ACTION PLAN FOR

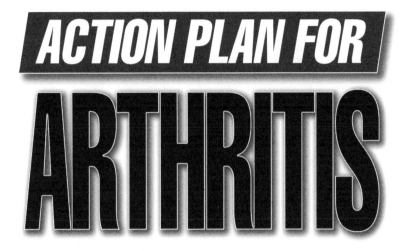

ARTHRITIS

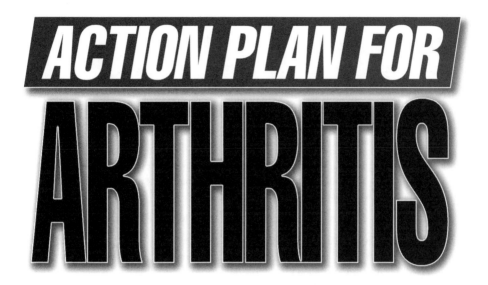

ACTION PLAN FOR ARTHRITIS

A. LYNN MILLAR, PT, PhD

HUMAN KINETICS

Library of Congress Cataloging-in-Publication Data

Millar, A. Lynn, 1955-
   Action plan for arthritis / A. Lynn Millar.
       p. cm.
Includes bibliographical references and index.
   ISBN 0-7360-4651-8 (soft cover)
   1.   Arthritis--Exercise therapy--Popular works.   I. Title.
   RC933.M54 2003
   616.7'22062--dc21

                                                                                2003008456

ISBN: 0-7360-4651-8

The Web addresses cited in this text were current as of July 2003, unless otherwise noted.

Acquisitions Editor: Martin Barnard; **Developmental Editor:** Leigh LaHood; **Assistant Editor:** John Wentworth; **Copyeditor:** Kathy Knight Calder; **Proofreader:** Anne Meyer Byler; **Indexer:** Betty Frizzéll; **Permission Manager:** Toni Harte; **Graphic Designer:** Fred Starbird; **Graphic Artist:** Tara Welsch; **Art and Photo Manager:** Dan Wendt; **Cover Designer:** Jack W. Davis; **Photographer (interior):** Dan Wendt, unless otherise noted; **Illustrator:** Mic Greenberg; **Printer:** United Graphics

Human Kinetics books are available at special discounts for bulk purchase. Special editions or book excerpts can also be created to specification. For details, contact the Special Sales Manager at Human Kinetics.

Printed in the United States of America   10   9   8   7   6   5   4   3   2   1

Human Kinetics
Web site: www.HumanKinetics.com

United States: Human Kinetics
P.O. Box 5076
Champaign, IL 61825-5076
800-747-4457
e-mail: humank@hkusa.com

Canada: Human Kinetics
475 Devonshire Road Unit 100
Windsor, ON N8Y 2L5
800-465-7301 (in Canada only)
e-mail: orders@hkcanada.com

Europe: Human Kinetics
107 Bradford Road
Stanningley
Leeds LS28 6AT, United Kingdom
+44 (0) 113 255 5665
e-mail: hk@hkeurope.com

Australia: Human Kinetics
57A Price Avenue
Lower Mitcham, South Australia 5062
08 8277 1555
e-mail: liahka@senet.com.au

New Zealand: Human Kinetics
P.O. Box 105-231, Auckland Central
09-523-3462
e-mail: hkp@ihug.co.nz

This book is dedicated to my family;
your support and love keep me going.

CONTENTS

CHAPTER 1
LIVING AND THRIVING WITH ARTHRITIS   1

*G*et the basics on preparing a new program: consulting your doctor, preventing injury, setting goals, establishing your fitness baseline, and identifying your individual needs.

CHAPTER 2
DESIGNING AN EXERCISE PROGRAM   31

*L*earn about the components of physical fitness, exercise principles, ways to stimulate a training response, and how to use all of them in your program planning.

CHAPTER 3
ADDING AEROBIC ACTIVITY   49

*U*se basic guidelines and sample programs for many different activities and fitness levels to customize your own aerobic workouts.

CHAPTER 4
BUILDING STRENGTH   75

*D*evelop a strength program by integrating information on resistance training, training locations, assembling exercises into workouts, and necessary precautions.

PREFACE

This book is written for the person who has arthritis and either is planning to start exercising or already is exercising and wishes to modify an existing program. It may also be helpful to those who work with arthritis patients and want to pull together information from both a clinical and a scientific perspective. Numerous research studies pertain to people with arthritis, but wading through various publications and interpreting the findings can be an overwhelming task for someone who wants to exercise. This book assembles relevant information from various fields of research and summarizes the findings. However, a simple summary of research findings is not necessarily useful. The chief purpose of this book, therefore, is to identify helpful information and combine it with clinical experience.

ACKNOWLEDGMENTS

Thank you to Kip, Marge, and my father for your stories, as well as the numerous patients and friends throughout the years whom I have used as examples.

INTRODUCTION

Arthritis affects more than 43 million people, the majority of them over the age of 45, and is a leading cause of impaired functioning in adults. Numerous types of arthritis affect joints, muscles, and sometimes other bodily systems. In fact, the Arthritis Foundation notes that there are more than 100 types of arthritis, the most common being osteoarthritis, osteoporosis, and rheumatoid arthritis. Regardless of the type, arthritis can have a destructive impact on one's activities and lifestyle. It often saps energy and leaves a person feeling fatigued and weak. The most common problem, joint and muscle pain, affects the ability to do household chores, to walk, to play, and even to carry out simple procedures like getting dressed.

We often hear about "magic" cures—such and such a product will decrease your pain and increase your strength, or following these easy steps will eliminate the discomfort of arthritis. Unfortunately, there are no magic cures; if any existed, we would all hear about them very rapidly from friends and family. Some advertisers suggest that their program is the one that will relieve your pain and allow you to lead a normal life. Most of these claims focus on pain relief, which is often temporary.

With the prevailing emphasis on pain relief goes the misconception that one should not exercise if any pain is present. Although this concept is true in specific situations, lack of exercise often increases joint or muscle pain for those who have arthritis and at the same time intensifies stiffness. Increased stiffness leads to deterioration of the ability to perform everyday tasks, thus starting a vicious cycle of escalating pain and declining function. Arthritis patients need to understand both the types of pain and ways to manage that pain while staying active.

You may have attempted to dig up information to help you set up an exercise program or modify your existing program, because of the problems caused by your arthritis. With today's technology, however, the amount of information available can be overwhelming. It is also difficult to determine which sources of information are reliable or, in some cases, even to understand the research you find.

As a professor of physical therapy, I teach my students not only how to analyze published research, but more important, how to make it comprehensible and useful to patients. In this book, I try to employ that same process. The book is based on a comprehensive review of research pertinent to arthritis and exercise. I have tried to translate scientific findings into useable guidelines and combine them with practical suggestions about exercise. The purpose is to help you exercise safely and effectively, despite your arthritis. Finally, when little scientific information is available about a matter that may affect your ability to exercise, I relate anecdotal evidence that may apply to your situation.

The book is divided into eight chapters, with a list of additional resources and references at the end. The first chapter focuses on evaluating your fitness and identifying your personal limitations before you start exercising. It also points out resources to help you achieve your goals, such as proper equipment and exercise facilities. The next four chapters identify the traditional components of a training regimen, exercise principles related to each component, and sample programs for both beginners and those who wish to modify an existing program.

I describe in detail what you should be doing and call attention to a few problematic activities. In chapter 6, I discuss alternative exercise programs such as tai chi and aerobic classes. Chapter 7 addresses a central concern for most people who have arthritis—joint protection. In this chapter, I describe not only traditional methods of joint protection such as splints and shoes, but also less conventional aids like supplements and nutrition.

Finally, chapter 8 takes up special circumstances you might have to cope with—arthritic flare-ups, joint replacement surgery, traveling, and adverse weather. It is my hope that you can use this book to begin an exercise program if you have not been exercising regularly, or to modify an existing program that is not working well for you. Above all, I hope to encourage you to get out and exercise, safely and effectively.

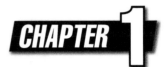

CHAPTER 1

LIVING AND THRIVING WITH ARTHRITIS

I could have titled this chapter "Dealing With Your Arthritis." I want to emphasize, however, that you can do more than just cope with the disease. You can thrive in spite of it. Do not view yourself as the victim of a problem—you are in control. The problems associated with arthritis do not simply disappear when you start exercising, but you no longer have to give up your life because of your arthritis. A good exercise program helps diminish the pain and disability associated with arthritis and allows you to enjoy some favorite activities. My grandmother was still living independently when she died at the age of 100. In fact, she walked several miles a day until her mid-90s, undeterred by her arthritis.

Some of you know that even pain in your hands significantly affects the things you can do and your outlook on life. I know of a woman whose arthritis in her hands became bad enough that she had to stop riding horses, her favorite pastime, because she could not hold the reins. She was caught in a vicious circle of decreasing activity and increasing pain, until her doctor diagnosed her problems as arthritis and she started an exercise program. She began a regular exercise program and now enjoys horseback riding and many other activities.

Types of Arthritis

Knowing about the type of arthritis you have and its causes and symptoms can help you best determine your exercise goals and plans. Arthritis is defined as inflammation of a joint, but it often affects more than just the joint, sometimes compromising the tissues that surround a joint and affecting other bodily systems.

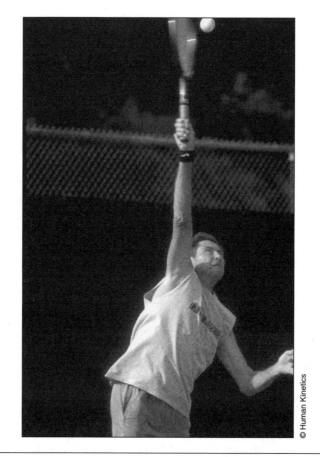

© Human Kinetics

Arthritis doesn't have to stop you from leading a full and active life.

Within the joint, the primary tissue affected is the articular cartilage. This tissue covers each inner part of most joints; it helps to disperse forces at the joint surface and allows for smooth movement of the joint. Loss or irregularities of this cartilage can increase friction within the joint; this is the main manifestation of *osteoarthritis*. A special lubricant called synovial fluid is produced within the joint that decreases normal friction and allows the surfaces to glide easily. This process is similar to oil allowing a hinge to move smoothly. Alteration in synovial fluid production is one of the early effects of *rheumatoid arthritis*.

Osteoarthritis

Osteoarthritis, the most common form of arthritis, accounts for more than 85 percent of arthritis cases. Osteoarthritis is a degenerative disease that affects the hip, knee, back, and hand joints, as well as others. The causes of osteoarthritis are numerous and can include trauma or infection, but often no cause is identifiable. Mechanical stress, combined with abnormal biomechanics, leads to the initial damage to the joint cartilage, which then starts to break down. Immobilization of a joint, such as being in a cast, can also lead to degenerative articular cartilage changes. Repetitive loading and unloading of the joint forces fluid into and out of the joint, getting nutrition to the articular cartilage. When a joint is immobilized, these compressive forces are absent. As damage to the articular cartilage progresses, the joint space lessens and the bone underlying the cartilage experiences abnormal stresses and deforms.

Doctors diagnose osteoarthritis by correlating a patient's history and physical examination to his or her x-ray and laboratory test results. The amount of joint damage is only predictive of severity of symptoms for a small part of the population, however. Risk factors include female gender, obesity, joint injury, occupation, and smoking.

Osteoarthritis symptoms can develop slowly or rapidly, depending on the cause of the arthritis, presence of other diseases, activity level, and other influences. For the majority of individuals, however, development of symptoms is gradual and slow. The most common complaint is aching within a joint, accompanied by stiffness after sitting for prolonged periods. This stiffness generally lasts less than 30 minutes and is resolved with gentle movement. Many patients report grating with movement of the involved joint, and as the disease progresses, the joint may become deformed and lose motion. As osteoarthritis results from articular cartilage damage, it may be limited to only one joint and, as noted earlier, occurs largely in the weight-bearing joints.

Rheumatoid Arthritis

Rheumatoid arthritis is the second most common joint disease, affecting approximately one to two percent of the adult population, though it can occur at any age. The cause of rheumatoid arthritis is not known, though two primary risk factors are age and female gender. The wrist, knee, hand, and foot joints are most affected. Rheumatoid arthritis is systemic in nature and thus affects tissues throughout the body, with joint involvement being bilateral. Changes in the synovial tissue alter synovial fluid production and ultimately damage the cartilage, bone, and adjacent tissues. Most of the extra-articular tissue changes occur over the long term, though some systemic symptoms are present from the onset.

Symptoms of rheumatoid arthritis usually start slowly and may be systemic complaints such as fatigue, weight loss, weakness, and general joint pain. In contrast to the stiffness felt with osteoarthritis, stiffness with rheumatoid arthritis lasts for more than 30 minutes. One criterion for diagnosis is morning stiffness that lasts at least an hour. Patients will often have periods during which their symptoms are worse, called exacerbations—the involved joints may be swollen, warm, and painful. As with osteoarthritis, the joint becomes deformed and loses motion as the disease progresses. Joints are more likely to become unstable with rheumatoid arthritis than with osteoarthritis, perhaps because of the changes in the tissues outside the joint. Because it is systemic, rheumatoid arthritis can affect the heart, lungs, and gastrointestinal systems, among others.

Spondyloarthropathies

Spondyloarthropathies are a group of arthritic diseases that do not fit into the previous two classifications. Ankylosing spondylitis, Reiter's syndrome, and psoriatic arthritis are the most common arthropathies, with ankylosing spondylitis being the most prevalent—it affects one to two percent of the population. The causes of ankylosing spondylitis are unknown, though risk factors include male gender, age, Caucasian race, and family history. Like rheumatoid arthritis, ankylosing spondylitis is systemic and causes complications throughout the body, for example in the cardiac and pulmonary systems. Joints of the spine are primarily involved, with some unilateral involvement in other large joints. Inflammation occurs in other tissues, especially at ligamentous attachments. Initial symptoms are backache and stiffness, more so in the morning. The trunk and neck become symptomatic over time and the individual may also complain of weight loss, excessive fatigue, and fever.

As noted in the introduction, there are over 100 types of arthritis, with the three that I have outlined composing the bulk of the diagnoses. The joint pain and stiffness inherent with all types can be significantly reduced with regular exercise. In the next section I discuss the importance of working with your physician. Your doctor will identify not only what type of arthritis you have, but also issues related to your personal arthritis history, which will determine the type of program you pursue.

Working With Your Physician

Before starting a new exercise program, consult your physician. It is rare for doctors to advise their patients not to exercise at all, but they may restrict the type of activity because of preexisting joint damage or other disease. Consulting your doctor is especially important if you have not had a recent physical exam. Information from the checkup will enable your doctor to answer some of your questions about beginning an exercise program. Many people think that they do not need to see a physician because they are feeling fine; however, many chronic diseases associated with aging develop slowly, without noticeable signs or symptoms.

I used to work in a clinic that carried out health screenings for corporations. One gentleman told us that he had started a fitness program on his own the year before but had not been to a physician for years. Unfortunately, his stress test revealed significant coronary abnormalities, and he had to have bypass surgery the next day. Although the heart problem was identified and treated successfully, the lesson is this: Don't assume anything. Your physician will review your health history, age, current symptoms, and signs of developing problems and will determine whether you need any tests to complete your physical.

Approach the meeting with your physician as an informed and active participant, just as you take charge of your health by exercising. Find out what screening tests are generally recommended for your age and sex, and discuss with your physician the possible need for these tests. I also suggest making a list of questions to ask during your checkup and a list of any problems that you have had since you last saw a physician.

Communicate clearly and completely with your doctor. Most health care workers can tell stories about diagnoses that were initially missed because the patient either thought a problem was not worth mentioning or forgot to mention it. I treated a patient who was referred for a torn rotator cuff (shoulder muscle). As I talked to him, I kept thinking that his symptoms were not all consistent with the diagnosis. When I examined his shoulder, one of the first things I noticed was a large, blistery rash under the arm on that side. He said that his physician had not seen the rash, nor had he told the doctor about it; he did not think it was important. After a few tests I sent him back to his doctor, because the problem was not a rotator cuff tear but a systemic problem. Let your physician decide what is important, as doctors are trained to do.

Questions to Ask Your Physician

▷ What general precautions should I be aware of regarding exercise and my current health?

▷ Do any medications I take affect my ability to exercise or my response to exercise?

▷ Are there any activities that I should not do?

▷ Is my arthritis systemic or nonsystemic?

▷ Do I need to use a splint or other joint protection device to participate in the activity?

You need the answers to these questions before you start exercising, for several reasons. First, very few people over the age of 40 have only one health problem. The risk of having more than one disease at the same time increases with age, and people with arthritis have an increased risk of heart disease. You may have a health concern that is more important than your arthritis in determining exercise limitations, either because of the condition itself or because of the medication used to control it. The presence of some diseases contraindicates exercise or requires precautions that your doctor can identify. With some diseases, such as diabetes, doctors must know what exercise you plan to do so that they can monitor your response and adjust your medications when necessary. Even if you are not yet 40, your physician may want to screen you for the many systemic diseases than can start at a younger age. See table 1.1 for risk factors for arthritis.

Table 1.1   Risk Factors for Arthritis

Modifiable	Non-modifiable
Obesity	Age
Trauma	Previous injury
Muscular weakness	Gender

Second, the medications that you take may affect your ability to exercise or the way your body responds to exercise. For example, some of the most common medications used to control high blood pressure are beta-blockers. Beta-blockers affect your blood pressure and heart rate both at rest and during exercise. For this reason you may not be able to use heart rate to determine the intensity of aerobic exercise; you will need to use one of the other methods identified in chapter 3. Your doctor needs to know everything that you are taking, including supplements. Some herbal supplements and even some vitamins can interfere with the effectiveness of certain medications.

Finally, you need information about your specific type of arthritis, which will influence the activities you choose and the parameters of that activity. As noted in the introduction, there are more than 100 types of arthritis; some are systemic and some are specific to one or two joints. Your doctor can tell you which type you have and whether there are any contraindications to exercise or any special requirements for activities.

For example, rheumatoid arthritis affects numerous systems. People with this type of arthritis may need a lower-intensity activity, especially during flare-ups. Some arthritis patients need a protective device for a joint, such as a wrist or finger splint for activities involving the upper extremities. Your physician may have you see a physical therapist for a detailed musculoskeletal exam to determine the need for splints. You may also benefit from a prescription medication for pain and inflammation control. See table 1.2 for more examples of modifications for specific problems.

Injury Prevention

Once you have met with your physician, you are ready to plan or modify your program. Before you start exercising, be sure to review the key practices for preventing injury (I will also discuss most of these recom-

Table 1.2 Examples of Activity Modifications for Common Health Problems

Problem	Activity modifications
Joint inflammation	Lower impact; decrease range and intensity
Long-term steroid use	Lower impact
Low bone density	Lower impact
Cardiac disease	Monitor heart rate and blood pressure response
Diabetes	Lower impact; monitor responses

mendations in more detail in later chapters, although not necessarily in relation to injury prevention). Nothing you do will completely rule out the possibility of injury, but you can try to eliminate several predictors of injury.

Injuries are commonly classified as either traumatic or overuse injuries. Traumatic injuries during exercise include sprained joints, muscle strains, contusions, and broken bones. Unless you plan to participate in a vigorous group sport such as soccer, you probably do not need to worry about the last two. On the other hand, since most females start losing bone density during their 30s (men start losing density a little later), they do need to be concerned about fractures. Overuse injuries include stress fractures (a potential problem if you have low bone density) and tendinitis.

One predictor of injury is a history of injuries to particular body tissues, perhaps because the tissues involved do not completely return to their preinjury condition. Furthermore, an injury to the knee joint (or to a muscle that supports the knee) inhibits knee extensor strength, and this strength loss persists long after the injury has healed (Suter and Herzog 2000). The pathological changes that take place in tissues because of arthritis and aging increase a person's susceptibility to injury. The composition of cartilage changes, both in bones and in joints, and the joint capsule itself changes. These changes may cause instability in a joint and gradual loss of motion in the joint capsule (Hertling and Kessler 1996; Stamford 1988). The slow loss of muscular strength that occurs with aging also diminishes stability.

A special concern with arthritis is rest—or lack of it, which can contribute to both types of injury. Studies have shown that general fatigue is a factor in traumatic injuries, possibly caused by impaired reactions and poor decision making. Muscular fatigue may contribute to injury when it slows the force and speed of muscle contractions. Muscular and general fatigue often increases during arthritic flare-ups. I will discuss the importance of rest again later; it is a vital component of injury prevention.

Traumatic Injuries

Although most traumatic injuries are accidents, people can modify many elements that can contribute to such injuries. These contributors include unsuitable environment, poor equipment, inadequate warm-up, and lack of previous conditioning.

Exercising on a rocky or uneven surface increases the chance of ankle sprains or even dangerous falls, whereas there is less chance of such problems occurring on even ground. Proprioception, the ability to perceive a joint's position, decreases both after an injury to the knee and because of osteoarthritis (Hurley et al. 1997). This change in proprioception means that a person's response to an unexpected change in the exercise surface may be impaired, resulting in a fall. To worsen the situation, the muscles in the anterior thigh (quadriceps) are often inhibited because of previous injury or the effects of arthritis, decreasing their responsiveness. Keep to even surfaces when you begin your program. The good news is that a regular exercise program results in improved muscular function and balance.

Shoes that fit poorly or do not give adequate support also increase the chance of injury. Watch the movement of a woman's ankle when she is walking in heels and you will see side-to-side rocking. The same type of movement occurs in a shoe that fits poorly or does not have a good supportive base, though it is not as noticeable. Such excess movement increases the potential for ankle sprains and foot pain.

Lack of warm-up often leads to muscle strains, to which you may already be more susceptible because of your arthritis. Both arthritis and aging make tissues less elastic and more brittle. If a sudden strain is put on such tissues, they are more prone to tear. A good warm-up increases blood flow and tissue temperature in the exercising muscles, which increases the elasticity of the tissues involved. The warm-up also increases neural stimulation to the active muscles, perhaps improving their responsiveness to unusual stresses.

Finally, your level of conditioning, especially muscular conditioning, can affect your susceptibility to injury. Muscle weakness in the lower extremities may result in poor balance, and pain from osteoarthritis may accentuate this problem (Jadelis et al. 2001). As mentioned earlier, conditioning also improves joint proprioception, which works with muscles to react to balance changes.

Overuse Injuries

Most clinicians agree that younger people are more prone to traumatic injuries, whereas older people tend to have a greater percentage of overuse problems. Of course, both groups get both types of injuries. The difference may be due to the biological changes that slowly occur in joints and tissues, as well as the type of activities different age groups participate in. Some of the tissue changes that occur with arthritis, especially during the inflammatory stages, are similar to those of aging—loss of fluid, decreased elasticity, and increased susceptibility to tearing (Buckwalter and Mankin 1997). The cartilage that covers joint surfaces becomes vulnerable to injury caused by tissue fatigue, which is further aggravated by lack of blood flow to the inner parts of that tissue (Hertling and Kessler 1996). Overuse injuries are related to improper equipment and exercise progression, as well as an imbalanced exercise program.

Shoes that do not provide proper support or good cushioning for the feet are a common contributor to overuse injuries. Lack of support or cushioning affects the way force is transmitted throughout the lower extremities. Shoes that allow excessive movement at the ankle are connected to knee pain, and correction of the shoes can significantly ease the pain (Hanes 1996).

Advancing your program too rapidly has been identified as one of the biggest predictors of overuse injuries, in part because of problems caused by an imbalanced program. As I discuss in the next chapter, a slow progression allows your bones and tissues time to adapt to the new stresses that unaccustomed exercise places on them. Gains in strength take time, and lack of strength around a joint can increase the stress that is transmitted to ligaments and bones, which increases the chance of an overuse reaction. An imbalanced program has a similar effect. Inadequate strength or flexibility in an area may lead to poor biomechanics and possible injury.

Importance of Rest

An important consideration for people with arthritis is getting the proper balance between exercise and rest. Just as you need exercise to maintain function and enjoy diverse activities, you also require adequate rest. In fact, you need two types of rest—general and joint-specific (Minor and Westby 2001).

Arthritis, especially in the lower extremities, alters one's biomechanics during walking and other activities. With changes in biomechanics, the body expends more energy to perform simple chores and thus fatigues more rapidly. Focus on getting a full night's sleep—which may be six hours for some people, nine for others—so that you feel rested in the morning. Also, incorporate short morning and afternoon rest periods into your routine. A friend said she used to feel guilty about needing a regular short rest period when she came home from work, until the doctor told her that the rest periods were an important part of her routine. A regular rest routine helps protect other bodily systems and is crucial during arthritis flare-ups.

Joint-specific rest is necessary for joints that are compromised and may be inflamed. During inflammation, the joints are usually less stable and at greater risk for injury. Joint rest involves decreased loading on that joint, which you can accomplish in several ways. For lower-extremity joints, alter the exercise to reduce the amount of impact and decrease the movement stresses applied to the joint. For example, you may choose cycling rather than jogging until inflammation subsides. You can also splint a joint to protect it during this time of increased vulnerability. Both general and joint-specific rest are components of injury prevention, because they allow the tissues to respond properly when needed. In chapter 8, I will point out potential indicators of overuse and lack of rest and discuss what to do in response.

Setting Goals

Once the doctor clears you to start exercising, you are ready to move ahead. Behavioralists suggest that people go through several stages to change, and that the activities you participate in may help to move you from one stage to the next (Prochaska and DiClemente 1982). If you have not been exercising but are thinking about starting a program, you are in the *contemplation* stage. Two activities that will help you move to the next stage are education, which you are doing by reading this book, and analyzing your current activity level. The next stage of change is *preparation*, during which you take the initial steps toward the intended change. During this stage you should define your exercise goals (or redefine them if you are already exercising). This step helps you to determine the extent of the program you design and to stay motivated, especially during the first few weeks of your program. Hoeger and Hoeger suggest writing down your goals, because "an unwritten goal is simply a wish" (2002, p. 38).

Make sure that your goals are realistic and, at least in part, objective. A broad, vague goal such as "get fit" gives you nothing concrete by which you can measure your accomplishments. Think about what "getting fit" means to you; is it being able to walk nine holes of golf easily, carry your groceries from the car to the house, or lose weight? We may all start with vague, general goals; but when we think about it, there is usually something specific that we want to achieve. Identify the more specific goal; you may even find that you have several related goals. A golfer may want to increase her endurance (decrease fatigue during a round) and gain more shoulder flexibility to improve her golf swing.

Long-Term Goals

Long-term goals are those that you plan to achieve over several months or years. Set a long-term goal, then develop a specific short-term goal that works toward meeting the long-term objective. In the golfing example just mentioned, one can fine-tune the goal of decreasing fatigue during a round of golf: Be able to walk 18 holes at the pace needed to complete a round in

4 1/2 hours. Making the goal measurable enables you to identify the steps you must take to reach it and to determine whether you have indeed met your goal. The golfer's flexibility goal is achievable in the short term, but a good long-term goal might be to perform a regular shoulder-stretching routine on a daily basis.

After you identify your goal, check to make sure it is realistic. Find out whether others in your peer group can complete the round in the target time. If you were able to meet the goal at one time, you will have an idea of how feasible it is and how long you may take to achieve it. It will take longer to reach this goal if you have been driving a cart for the last year than if you are already able to walk 9 holes at a comfortable pace.

Short-Term Goals

After you have identified your long-term goals, divide them into short-term goals that cover perhaps 2 to 4 weeks. Some call these short-term goals objectives—the steps one takes to reach a goal. In the golfing example, one cannot make dramatic improvements in endurance in only 2 to 4 weeks. An intermediate long-term goal (reached in perhaps 3 months) can be to walk 9 holes at a comfortable pace. A short-term objective can be doing something toward that goal: Walk 2 times a day, for 10 minutes each time, at a moderate pace. You can further fine-tune this goal by using the information in the chapter on aerobics to determine the heart rate you should reach during your walks.

A person can achieve the goal of flexibility within a short-term period. The goal can read as follows: Achieve and maintain shoulder range of motion to within approximately 10 degrees of normal for all motions. Here is a less objective but still useful goal: Be able to point both arms toward the sky and touch the middle of the neck and back with each hand. Using methods described later, you can determine your baseline (starting level), for both shoulder flexibility and general endurance, and can then reevaluate each at an appropriate time. As you will see, the way you assess your baseline and response to exercise can range from very subjective to objective, depending on the type of feedback that is most helpful to you. Doing a baseline assessment will help you transition from the preparation stage to the third stage—*action*—during which an individual starts doing or modifies his or her behavior.

Regardless of your goals and method of measuring progress, there will be times when you do not make progress. You may reach a plateau or even have a small setback—especially as you get older and because of the intermittent nature of arthritis. People may joke about telling the weather by a specific joint, but it highlights the day-to-day variability that sometimes occurs with arthritis (as with some other diseases).

One young man told me he only has shoulder symptoms when it is damp outside. I have low back problems that sometimes flare up, causing pain in my thigh. During those times, I switch from jogging to walking and decrease the amount that I lift during my strength-training sessions. As the symptoms subside, I slowly progress back to jogging and increase my weights. My goals haven't changed, but my timeline for specific objectives sometimes needs to be adjusted. It is wise to listen to your body.

Establishing a Baseline

Each person has different approaches to attaining goals, but some common steps are helpful. One of the first steps is establishing your baseline—that is, your starting capabilities for each goal. If you want to decrease your fatigue while walking, you must establish how far you can currently walk without fatigue. Measuring your baseline can be simple or complex, depending on your need. If you have not been exercising at all, I recommend a slightly more comprehensive baseline test—although none of the tests identified here are extremely complicated. If you are already active but wish to modify your program, you may only do a formal test for new areas or the ones you want to modify.

For example, if you walk regularly but have realized that you need to add some resistance training, do baseline tests for strength. For your walking routine, note your current fitness level using the distance of the walk or the duration and intensity of the routine. Regardless of your level, you need to have some idea of your initial fitness status, both for determining the initial program and for tracking progress. As I will discuss in chapter 2, there are three basic components of fitness—cardiovascular (aerobic) endurance, muscular strength, and flexibility.

Aerobic Fitness Tests

Aerobic fitness or endurance can be assessed using one of several tests. Most of the tests estimate oxygen consumption (abbreviated as $\dot{V}O_2max$), which is the physiological measure of aerobic fitness. Your physician may have you do a treadmill stress test, which provides an accurate baseline for aerobic fitness. Otherwise, test yourself to establish your baseline. Select a test that reflects the activity you currently do or plan to do; for example, if you intend to start a cycling program, measure your baseline fitness using a bicycle test. You can choose from some of the easiest, most common field tests for a variety of activities, descriptions of which follow.

Immediately before a test, warm up with some gentle activities that raise your heart rate and make you feel limber. Walking in place for a few minutes or cycling without resistance is a good way to loosen up your legs. If you are going to do the swimming test, stretch your shoulders and trunk using some easy shoulder circles and trunk bends and twists. For any of the tests, you have to make a good effort for the results to be meaningful.

You also need to know how to take your pulse for several of the tests. If you have never taken your heart rate, it is easiest to take using the pulse at your wrist (radial pulse). The best way to take your pulse is to use the index and middle fingers of the opposite hand (see figure 1.1). Do not use your thumb—it has its own pulse and will give you an erroneous count. The pulse is located between two tendons of the wrist, at the base of your thumb. Using a gentle pressure, you should be able to feel the pulse. I suggest practicing several times before performing an exercise test.

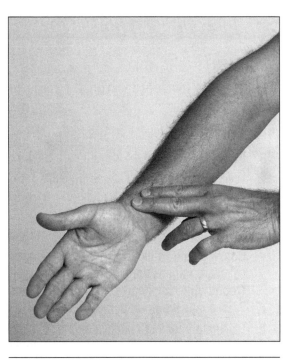

Figure 1.1 Taking radial pulse.

Walking Test

The Rockport Walk Test has been validated with healthy adults and is probably an easier test to complete than some of the other walking and jogging tests, such as the 12-minute run test (Dolgener et al. 1994; Kline et al. 1987). The Rockport test involves walking a mile for time and gives an estimate of your aerobic fitness using the total time and your heart rate, gender, and weight. The results are plugged into a formula that calculates oxygen consumption. As fitness improves, your mile time will decrease. See page 14 for this test.

Cycling Test

If you plan to cycle or swim as your aerobic activity, select a test specific to those activities. The Åstrand bike test, detailed on pages 15-18, is simple to perform; it relies on increasing the resistance of pedaling, so you may find it uncomfortable (Åstrand and Rhyming 1954). Cycle at a predetermined resistance for 6 minutes, taking your heart rate every minute. Because of the need to take your heart rate during the test, it may be easier to have someone help you. Your oxygen consumption is then calculated using a nomogram, which you adjust for age (Åstrand 1960).

▷ 1-Mile Walk Test (Rockport Walk Test)

EQUIPMENT

400-meter track (outdoor track) or other measured course, a stopwatch, and a weight scale

PROCEDURE

1. Measure body weight to the nearest pound.
2. Walk 1.0 mile as quickly as possible, noting your total time to complete the mile.
3. At the end of the mile, immediately take your pulse for 10 seconds. Multiply this number by 6 to obtain your heart rate in beats per minute (bpm).
4. Convert your walking time from minutes and seconds to minute units. To calculate minute units, divide the number of seconds by 60 to get a fraction (round up to the nearest hundredth). Thus, a walking time of 15 minutes and 37 seconds would become 15 + (37/60) = 15.62.
5. Calculate your estimated maximal oxygen consumption ($\dot{V}O_2$max) using the following formula, then use table 1.5 to determine your fitness classification.

$$\dot{V}O_2\text{max in ml/kg/min} = 132.853 - (0.0769 \times W) - (0.3877 \times A) + (6.315 \times G) - (3.2649 \times T) - (0.1565 \times HR)$$

W = weight in pounds

A = age in years

G = gender (0 = female; 1 = male)

T = total converted time, in minutes

HR = heart rate in bpm for 1.0 mile walk

EXAMPLE

You are a 49-year-old female, with a weight of 145 pounds. Your time for the walk was 16 minutes and 42 seconds, and your 10-second pulse was 23.

$$T = 16 + 42/60 = 16.7 \qquad HR = 23 \times 6 = 138 \text{ bpm}$$

$$\dot{V}O_2\text{max} = 132.853 - (0.0769 \times 145) - (0.3877 \times 49) + (6.315 \times 0) - (3.2649 \times 16.7) - (0.1565 \times 138)$$

$$= 132.853 - 11.1505 - 18.9973 + 0 - 54.52383 - 21.597$$

$$\dot{V}O_2\text{max} = 26.6 \text{ ml/kg/min}$$

Adapted, by permission, from Kline et al. 1987.

EQUIPMENT

Stationary cycle with adjustable, measured resistance; stopwatch; and weight scale

PROCEDURE

1. Measure body weight to nearest pound and convert to kilograms (abbreviated as kg; weight in pounds divided by 2.2046).

2. Adjust bicycle seat; at the bottom of the pedal revolution, your knees should be almost completely straight.

3. Start pedaling, increasing speed to 50 revolutions per minute. Maintaining this speed throughout the test, increase the resistance to the recommended level (consider your age and health; if you are older or in poorer health, select the lower of the two levels):

	Females	Males
Unconditioned	300 or 450 kpm	300 or 600 kpm
Conditioned	450 or 600 kpm	600 or 900 kpm

4. Start the stopwatch, continuing pedal cadence for 6 minutes. Check your heart rate for the last 10 seconds of each minute. Convert each 10-second count to heart rate in bpm by multiplying each count by 6.

5. If the last two minutes (5 and 6) are within 5 beats of each other, average them to get your test heart rate. If they are not, continue for a few minutes until they are within 5 beats of each other. If your heart rate continues to increase greatly after the sixth minute, stop the test and rest for approximately 15 minutes. You may then perform the test again at the next lower workload. Your final average heart rate should be from 120 to 140 bpm for the lower workloads and from 120 to 170 for the higher workloads.

6. Using the final averaged heart rate, find your $\dot{V}O_2$max (l/min) in table 1.3, then correct this value for age using the numbers found in table 1.4.

7. To find $\dot{V}O_2$max in ml/kg/min, complete the following calculations:

$$\dot{V}O_2\text{max in ml/kg/min} = \frac{\text{l/min} \times 1{,}000}{\text{Weight (kg)}}$$

8. Using oxygen consumption value, find fitness classification in table 1.5.

EXAMPLE

You are a 67-year-old male, unconditioned, with a weight of 195 pounds. You complete the test at 300 kpm, with an average heart rate of 132 bpm.

$$\dot{V}O_2max \ (l/min) = 1.8$$
$$\dot{V}O_2max \ (l/min) \text{ age corrected} = .65 \times 1.8 = 1.17$$
$$Weight = 88.5 \text{ kg}$$
$$\dot{V}O_2max \text{ in ml/kg/min} = \frac{1.17 \times 1,000}{88.5} = 13.2 \text{ ml/kg/min}$$

Reprinted, by permission, from Åstrand 1960.

Table 1.3   Åstrand-Rhyming Bicycle Test—Oxygen Consumption Rates Based on Workload and Heart Rate

Heart rate	Workload for men					Workload for women				
	300	600	900	1200	1500	300	450	600	750	900
120	2.2	3.4	4.8			2.6	3.4	4.1	4.8	
121	2.2	3.4	4.7			2.5	3.3	4.0	4.8	
122	2.2	3.4	4.6			2.5	3.2	3.9	4.7	
123	2.1	3.4	4.6			2.4	3.1	3.9	4.6	
124	2.1	3.3	4.5	6.0		2.4	3.1	3.8	4.5	
125	2.0	3.2	4.4	5.9		2.3	3.0	3.7	4.4	
126	2.0	3.2	4.4	5.8		2.3	3.0	3.6	4.3	
127	2.0	3.1	4.3	5.7		2.2	2.9	3.5	4.2	
128	2.0	3.1	4.2	5.6		2.2	2.8	3.5	4.2	4.8
129	1.9	3.0	4.2	5.6		2.2	2.8	3.4	4.1	4.8
130	1.9	3.0	4.1	5.5		2.1	2.7	3.4	4.0	4.7
131	1.9	2.9	4.0	5.4		2.1	2.7	3.4	4.0	4.6
132	1.8	2.9	4.0	5.3		2.0	2.7	3.3	3.9	4.5

Heart rate	Workload for men					Workload for women				
	300	600	900	1200	1500	300	450	600	750	900
133	1.8	2.8	3.9	5.3		2.0	2.6	3.2	3.8	4.4
134	1.8	2.8	3.9	5.2		2.0	2.6	3.2	3.8	4.4
135	1.7	2.8	3.8	5.1		2.0	2.6	3.1	3.7	4.3
136	1.7	2.7	3.8	5.0		1.9	2.5	3.1	3.6	4.2
137	1.7	2.7	3.7	5.0		1.9	2.5	3.0	3.6	4.2
138	1.6	2.7	3.7	4.9		1.8	2.4	3.0	3.5	4.1
139	1.6	2.6	3.6	4.8		1.8	2.4	2.9	3.5	4.0
140	1.6	2.6	3.6	4.8	6.0	1.8	2.4	2.8	3.4	4.0
141		2.6	3.5	4.7	5.9	1.8	2.3	2.8	3.4	3.9
142		2.5	3.5	4.6	5.8	1.7	2.3	2.8	3.3	3.9
143		2.5	3.4	4.6	5.7	1.7	2.2	2.7	3.3	3.8
144		2.5	3.4	4.5	5.7	1.7	2.2	2.7	3.2	3.8
145		2.4	3.4	4.5	5.6	1.6	2.2	2.7	3.2	3.7
146		2.4	3.3	4.4	5.6	1.6	2.2	2.6	3.2	3.7
147		2.4	3.3	4.4	5.5	1.6	2.1	2.6	3.1	3.6
148		2.4	3.2	4.3	5.4	1.6	2.1	2.6	3.1	3.6
149		2.3	3.2	4.3	5.4		2.1	2.6	3.0	3.5
150		2.3	3.2	4.2	5.3		2.0	2.5	3.0	3.5
151		2.3	3.1	4.2	5.2		2.0	2.5	3.0	3.4
152		2.3	3.1	4.1	5.2		2.0	2.5	2.9	3.4
153		2.2	3.0	4.1	5.1		2.0	2.4	2.9	3.3
154		2.2	3.0	4.0	5.1		2.0	2.4	2.8	3.3

(continued)

Table 1.3 *(continued)*

Heart rate	Workload for men					Workload for women				
	300	600	900	1200	1500	300	450	600	750	900
155		2.2	3.0	4.0	5.0		1.9	2.4	2.8	3.2
156		2.2	2.9	4.0	5.0		1.9	2.3	2.8	3.2
157		2.1	2.9	3.9	4.9		1.9	2.3	2.7	3.2
158		2.1	2.9	3.9	4.9		1.8	2.3	2.7	3.1
159		2.1	2.8	3.8	4.8		1.8	2.2	2.7	3.1
160		2.1	2.8	3.8	4.8		1.8	2.2	2.6	3.0
161		2.0	2.8	3.7	4.7		1.8	2.2	2.6	3.0
162		2.0	2.8	3.7	4.6		1.8	2.2	2.6	3.0
163		2.0	2.8	3.7	4.6		1.7	2.2	2.6	2.9
164		2.0	2.7	3.6	4.5		1.7	2.1	2.5	2.9
165		2.0	2.7	3.6	4.5		1.7	2.1	2.5	2.9
166		1.9	2.7	3.6	4.5		1.7	2.1	2.5	2.8
167		1.9	2.6	3.5	4.4		1.6	2.1	2.4	2.8
168		1.9	2.6	3.5	4.4		1.6	2.0	2.4	2.8
169		1.9	2.6	3.5	4.3		1.6	2.0	2.4	2.8
170		1.8	2.6	3.4	4.3		1.6	2.0	2.4	2.7

Reprinted, by permission, from Åstrand 1960.

Swimming Test

A 12-minute swim test for distance exists that gives an estimate of your fitness level (Hoeger and Hoeger 2002; Cooper 1982). I usually suggest this test only if you are already swimming and do not have arthritis in your shoulders, for two reasons. First, if you have not been swimming, you may find that this test aggravates your shoulder symptoms. Second, although you may have been working out, unless you have been training your shoulders you may have difficulty swimming for 12 minutes continuously. On the other hand, if you have not been swimming, you should see

Table 1.4   Age Correction Factors

Age	Correction factor	Age	Correction factor
20	1.05	43	.800
21	1.04	44	.790
22	1.03	45	.780
23	1.02	46	.774
24	1.01	47	.768
25	1.00	48	.762
26	.987	49	.756
27	.974	50	.750
28	.961	51	.742
29	.948	52	.734
30	.935	53	.726
31	.922	54	.718
32	.909	55	.710
33	.896	56	.704
34	.883	57	.698
35	.870	58	.692
36	.862	59	.686
37	.854	60	.680
38	.846	61	.674
39	.838	62	.668
40	.830	63	.662
41	.820	64	.656
42	.810	65	.650

Reprinted, by permission, from Åstrand 1960.

significant improvement once you get started. The distance you cover during the 12-minute period is used to identify a fitness category.

I suggest that you determine your baseline for swimming in one of two ways: swim as many laps as you can in 10 minutes and use that distance as your baseline, or record the total number of laps you are able swim continuously and work on improving that.

Refining Your Aerobic Goal

The various test results will give you either a fitness classification, such as "fair," or an estimate of oxygen consumption, which is the physiological measure. If the results are given as an estimate of oxygen consumption, you can convert the estimate to a fitness category. The fitness classifications for oxygen consumption values are given in table 1.5. Use this baseline measure to refine your goals.

For example, if you use the walking test and find that your fitness level is in the "fair" category, then your long-term goal might be to advance your cardiovascular fitness to the next category, "good." Your short-term goal might be to decrease your walking time for the mile walk by 30 seconds within 2 months. This sort of goal is very specific, and you will be able to see if you are making progress. I suggest that you also include a subjective evaluation—how you feel at the end of the mile test, in terms of both fatigue and symptoms. Sometimes it takes longer to reach the measurable goals for time, but you may find that your perception of fatigue or pain has lessened.

As I suggested, testing can be as simple or complex as you wish, so you can alter the tests to match your needs or capabilities. For walking, you

Table 1.5 Fitness Classification for Maximal Oxygen Consumption Values

| | Age | Fitness classification | | | | |
		Poor	Fair	Average	Good	Excellent
Men	≤29	≤35	36-40	41-45	46-50	≥51
	30-39	≤33	34-37	38-43	44-49	≥50
	40-49	≤31	32-35	36-40	41-47	≥48
	50-59	≤29	30-32	33-37	38-44	≥45
	60+	≤24	25-29	30-34	35-41	≥42
Women	≤29	≤28	29-32	33-37	38-43	≥44
	30-39	≤27	28-31	30-35	36-40	≥41
	40-49	≤25	26-28	29-32	33-38	≥39
	50-59	≤22	23-25	26-29	30-34	≥35
	60+	≤21	22-23	24-28	29-34	≥35

Adapted, by permission, from ACSM 2000.

can measure how many blocks you can cover in a specified time (total time should be at least 5 minutes) or how long it takes you to walk around your block. If you are cycling outdoors, see how far you can cycle in a given time, or perhaps how long it takes you to ride to a predetermined destination. A similar test works for swimming—find out how many laps you can swim without stopping. Whether you use an established test or one of your own, write it down and use the baseline measure to evaluate your progress.

I am a jogger and time myself on a course around the neighborhood to keep track of my cardiovascular fitness. I do not time myself every day, which can be especially discouraging if stiffness or other problems are flaring up, but I try to time myself every few months. I encourage you to do the same. As with goals, you may be less likely to forget reevaluating yourself if you determine a day and write it into your plan ahead of time.

Strength Tests

Strength baseline is usually established by measurement of a 1-repetition maximum (1RM) or 10-repetition maximum, which is how much weight you can lift only 1 or 10 times. As this test often requires the help of a professional, you may select some easier methods at home. I usually have patients who have not been doing anything start out with high-repetition, low-resistance activities and do a repetition maximum assessment later, after they are accustomed to some strengthening exercises. A timed curl-up test (American College of Sports Medicine 1995) is a good general measure of trunk strength and endurance. Likewise, you can get an estimate of upper-body strength and endurance using a push-up test. Both of these tests are simple, use only your body weight, and have age-related normative values. The tests are explained on pages 22 and 23.

To do a repetition maximum test for strength, decide whether you want a 1RM, 10RM, or some other protocol baseline. Next, decide what strength exercises you are going to use in your program, since you will do the RM test for each exercise. Although many formulas have been suggested for estimating the 1RM, none of them is perfect. The best way is to estimate a potential load based on your current activity, age, and body size. Having a fitness professional assist you is a good idea. Finding the RM is often a matter of trial and error. Estimate what you think you can lift that first time, then try it. If you can lift it easily, increase the weight; if you cannot move it at all, decrease the weight. If you are not good at estimating (or the fitness person is not), you may need to complete the test another day. A caution is in order here—if you do a lot of lifting that you are not used to, you may have muscle soreness and increased arthritis symptoms in the next day or two.

▷ Timed Curl-Up Test for Abdominal Strength

EQUIPMENT

Timer or counter

PROCEDURE

1. Lie on your back on the floor with your knees bent to approximately 100 degrees (feet flat on the floor).
2. Cross your arms over your chest, putting each hand on the opposite shoulder.
3. Raise your head off the floor, with chin on chest, and bring your body to an upright position, then lower back to the floor.
4. Complete as many repetitions as possible in a 1-minute period, having the timer count the number of completed curl-ups.
5. Compute fitness rating from table below.

	Age	Fitness classification				
		Very poor	Poor	Fair	Good	Excellent
Men	20-29	≤32	33-37	38-41	42-46	≥47
	30-39	≤30	30-33	35-37	39-42	≥43
	40-49	≤23	24-28	29-32	34-37	≥39
	50-59	≤18	19-22	24-27	28-33	≥35
	60+	≤14	15-18	19-21	22-28	≥30
Women	20-29	≤26	27-31	32-37	38-42	≥44
	30-39	≤19	20-24	25-28	29-33	≥35
	40-49	≤13	14-19	20-23	24-28	≥29
	50-59	≤9	10-12	14-19	20-22	≥24
	60+	≤2	3-5	6-10	11-15	≥17

Fitness classification reprinted, by permission, from ACSM 2000.

▷ Push-Up Test for Upper-Body and Trunk Strength

EQUIPMENT

Counter

PROCEDURE

1. Lie on the ground on your stomach and position your hands by your shoulders (palms down). Men will keep legs straight, with their feet as the lower contact point, while women will bend their knees to 90 degrees, using the knees as the lower contact point.
2. Push up until arms are fully extended, then lower the body toward the floor. When lowered, the chest should be no higher than four inches (a fist width) from the floor, but should not touch the floor between push-ups.
3. Your back must remain straight throughout the push-up.
4. Count the number of push-ups you complete without stopping (there is no time limit).
5. Using the chart below, calculate your fitness level.

	Age	Fitness classification				
		Very poor	Poor	Fair	Good	Excellent
Men	20-29	≤21	22-27	29-35	37-44	≥47
	30-39	≤16	17-21	24-29	30-36	≥39
	40-49	≤10	11-16	18-22	24-29	≥30
	50-59	≤8	9-11	13-17	19-24	≥25
	60+	≤5	6-9	10-16	18-22	≥23
Women	20-29	≤15	17-22	23-29	30-34	≥36
	30-39	≤10	11-17	19-23	24-29	≥31
	40-49	≤5	6-11	13-17	18-21	≥24
	50-59	≤5	6-10	12-15	17-20	≥21
	60+	≤1	2-4	5-11	12-15	≥16

Fitness classification reprinted, by permission, from ACSM 2000.

Flexibility Tests

Measurement of flexibility can be divided into general flexibility and specific flexibility. It is simpler to test flexibility if you have someone help you. Otherwise, you may need to resort to a more functional assessment, such as whether you can touch your toes without bending your knees. Two easy tests for general flexibility are the sit-and-reach test, which can be modified to do at home, and a combined shoulder movement test (ACSM 1995). The sit-and-reach test gives you some information about low back and hamstring flexibility, while the combined shoulder test evaluates multiple movements of the shoulder. I have modified a clinical test called the Apley's scratch test for combined shoulder movements and have identified some functional criteria for the test, since no normative data are available for it (see page 26). Therapists often use this test to screen for shoulder joint involvement (Hoppenfeld 1976).

Specific joint flexibility identifies the available range of a joint in each of the normal movements for that joint. For example, the shoulder joint (for which you can check general flexibility using the modified Apley's scratch test) performs flexion, extension, internal and external rotation, adduction, and abduction. Specific joint flexibility is best measured by a professional, but you can estimate it visually if necessary. Assess how much knee flexion you have by sitting on the edge of a chair and moving one foot back into flexion (toward your buttocks). If you consider completely straight as zero degrees, you can determine how many degrees you can attain without using your hands for assistance. You can then compare it to the other joint, or to someone with healthy joints, and determine if you need to work on that range. If flexibility is noticeably lacking in one area, your physician may refer you to a therapist. Many of us have some small deficits in motion, but they require assessment when function is affected—that is, when you cannot perform a specific task.

Again, the more concrete the baseline and your objectives, the easier it will be for you to monitor your progress. You might make a sheet that lists your baseline measures and your goals. It will aid you when you start designing your program, a process I cover in the next chapter. One way to improve adherence to an exercise program is to keep an exercise diary. You can begin with your baseline measures and objectives, then use the diary to keep track of your training sessions.

Identifying Your Needs

Once you set your goals, you are ready to build a training program to reach those goals. Before you can do so, determine what you need to start the program and to help you stick with it. Basic needs include equipment

▷ Modified Sit-and-Reach Test

EQUIPMENT

Helper; yardstick with masking tape indicating the 15-inch mark

PROCEDURE

1. Sit on the floor and place the yardstick between your legs. The zero end of the yardstick is turned toward your trunk and your heels are even with the 15-inch mark. Your legs are 10 to 12 inches apart (no shoes).
2. Place your hands over each other, with the fingertips even. Your knees should be as straight as possible.
3. The helper is responsible for helping to keep the knees straight without pressing down on them, holding the yardstick so it does not slide, and noting the distance reached to the nearest half-inch.
4. Reach gently and slowly as far along the yardstick as you can, while maintaining knee and hand positions. Do not bounce. You should be able to maintain your maximum distance comfortably, without holding your breath, while your helper records the distance in inches.
5. Repeat the sequence 3 times, using the best distance as your score.
6. Use the chart below to calculate your fitness classification.

	Age	Fitness classification				
		Very poor	Poor	Fair	Good	Excellent
Men	20-29	≤13.5	14-16	16.5-18	18.5-20	≥20.5
	30-39	≤12	13-15	15.5-17	17.5-19	≥19.5
	40-49	≤11	12-14	14.5-16	16.5-18	≥18.5
	50-59	≤10	10.5-12.5	13-15	15.5-17	≥17.5
	60+	≤9	10-12	12.5-14	14.5-16.5	≥17
Women	20-29	≤16.5	17-19	19.5-20	20.5-22	≥22.5
	30-39	≤15.5	16.5-18	18.5-19.5	20-21	≥21.5
	40-49	≤14	15-17	17.5-18.5	19-20	≥20.5
	50-59	≤14	15-16	16.5-18	18.5-20	≥20.5
	60+	≤11.5	13-15	15.5-17	17-18	≥19

Fitness classification reprinted, by permission, from ACSM 2000.

▷ Combined Shoulder Flexibility Test (Modified Apley Scratch Test)

EQUIPMENT

Observer

PROCEDURE

1. Reach one hand back over your shoulder, trying to reach as low as possible on the spine. The observer notes the final position.
2. Then bring the hand behind your lower back, reaching as far up spine as possible, while the observer again notes the final position.
3. Repeat with the other arm.

Classification	Upper arm	Lower arm
Excellent	Reaches below base of neck	Reaches above level of bottom of scapula
Good	Reaches back of neck	Reaches to level of bottom of scapula
Fair	Reaches side of neck	Reaches middle of low back
Poor	Cannot reach side of neck	Cannot reach middle of low back

and facilities, and may include classes, exercise partners, and community resources.

A good first step is to identify what facilities and equipment are available to you, which will help set some of the parameters of your exercise program. For instance, if there is a nearby YMCA with an arthritis aquatic program, you may decide to use that program for part of your aerobic regimen. I discuss other potential resources later in the book, but each community varies in the type and availability of resources.

To go back to a previous example, the golfer does not need much equipment to work on shoulder flexibility and so can do it at home. To improve endurance for walking nine holes of golf, however, a golfer has to walk or jog. If I were working with this person, I would ask questions such as, "Can you walk in your neighborhood? If so, will you?" or, "Are you more likely to stick with a walking or jogging program if you do it on a treadmill?" If a person wants to do a treadmill program, then is a treadmill available, either at home or in a nearby facility? I emphasize nearby, since one of the most common reasons cited by people for dropping out of an exercise program is inconvenience—either of getting to the facility or of getting into it and using the equipment. Sometimes a facility is available, but upon closer investigation you find that it is costly or constantly crowded. If you happen to be a senior, some facilities identify specific hours for seniors, during which time it may be less crowded.

Equipment needs vary, depending on your goals and the complexity of the program you design. For cardiovascular exercise, equipment can range from shoes to a treadmill. The most common apparatus used for aerobic exercise include treadmills, stationary cycles, and cross-country ski trainers. Some of the new devices on the market include elliptical trainers, stair steppers, and climbers. If you go to a facility, the site itself will determine the type of equipment you use. If you plan to buy equipment, you should try it out before you buy—some devices can cause increased lower-extremity symptoms. Knowing what to look for in a piece of equipment is important; some of the resources I have identified offer information about different apparatus. I will discuss the type of cardiovascular activities that I recommend in the next chapter.

An even wider range of equipment is available for resistance-training programs. At the simplest level, you need only your own body. Home program equipment can include elastic tubing, cuff weights, hand weights, and free weights. Some machines are available for home use, but people tend to use machines at facilities, because a greater assortment of exercises is available with the larger number of machines. The equipment in facilities also varies, so you need to pay close attention to what the place has to offer.

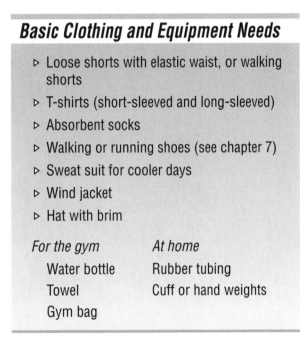

Basic Clothing and Equipment Needs

▷ Loose shorts with elastic waist, or walking shorts

▷ T-shirts (short-sleeved and long-sleeved)

▷ Absorbent socks

▷ Walking or running shoes (see chapter 7)

▷ Sweat suit for cooler days

▷ Wind jacket

▷ Hat with brim

For the gym	*At home*
Water bottle	Rubber tubing
Towel	Cuff or hand weights
Gym bag	

Support Mechanisms

Support mechanisms are resources that may help you achieve your goals. Examples are an exercise partner or someone who is willing to encourage you, childcare, arthritis support groups, or even classes. People often cite support from friends or family as a factor that encourages them to stick with their exercise programs. Family support can be as simple as scheduling dinner around your exercise time or as involved as participating in the exercise program with you.

Having an exercise partner is a great support mechanism. I have a friend who walks with another woman at 5:30 every morning before work. She says that when she knows someone will be waiting at the corner for her, she cannot talk herself out of exercising. Not only does she get exercise, but she enjoys the talks they have each day.

If you plan to exercise with someone, it is best if your abilities are similar. Otherwise it could be a good social time, but of little help in reaching your fitness goals. When I was first married, I thought my husband and I could start running together. I finally convinced him to go on a run with me during a vacation; at the end of the first mile I was gasping for air (probably the fastest mile I had ever done), when he asked if I was "warmed up yet." A good choice as a life partner, but not a good option as a training partner!

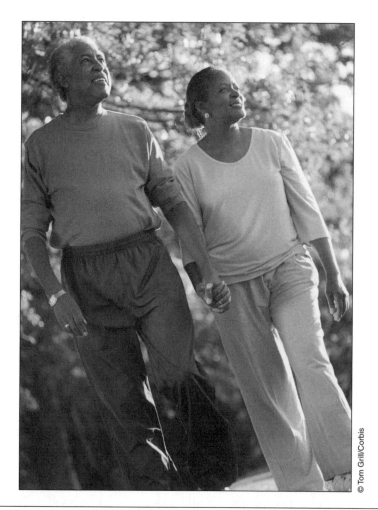

© Tom Grill/Corbis

Exercising with a friend or signing up for a walking or running event can give you motivation to stick with your program.

Perhaps you do not want to exercise with someone every day, but you like having social reinforcement. Find a group, or even a person, to meet with once a week for an exercise session. This arrangement combines social reinforcement with your desire to be more independent. Many areas have walking or running groups that meet once a week to exercise and socialize. Another way to build in social reinforcement is to enter local events. Entering an event does not mean you have to run. Many areas now have walking and cycling events, sometimes in conjunction with a running event or other health-related function. Even the goal of participating in an event can be reinforcing. Last summer my family had a large reunion, at the same time that the local community was having a 5K run and a 1K walk. It became a family event, with 10 of us competing in one of the two races. Several other families also participated in the races; the events provided lots of fun, exercise, and support.

After you determine where you want to go and where you currently are, you are ready to start designing an exercise program using that information. In chapter 2, I examine the components of fitness in more depth. I discuss what each component is, why it is important, and what some basic exercise principles are. It is my belief that the more you know, the more you are in control. You can make adjustments based on your needs, rather than following a "cookie-cutter" program.

ACTION PLAN:
PREPARING FOR A NEW PROGRAM

☐ Visit your doctor.

☐ Prevent injury in the following ways:

- Know your limitations.
- Understand the causes and types of injury.
- Get proper equipment (such as supportive shoes).
- Plan warm-ups and rest times.

☐ Set goals, both long-term and short-term.

☐ Establish your baseline through fitness, strength, and flexibility tests.

☐ Identify what keeps you from exercise and what encourages you to exercise.

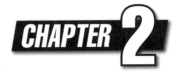

CHAPTER 2

DESIGNING AN EXERCISE PROGRAM

Y ou have decided to exercise, set some goals, and determined your baseline. Now you are ready to devise an exercise program that will help you reach your goals. You may currently be exercising and only wish to modify your routine to accommodate your arthritis. You may have reached this decision because you have trouble doing a specific activity, such as getting out of a chair or walking with your grandchild to the local park. You may think that you need to focus only on that activity, but if you only work on that one thing, you may not reach your goal. A gentleman that I know was trying to improve his ability to walk without fatigue but found that his knee pain was a major limiting factor. After starting a simple home strength program for his legs, he improved his ability to walk without pain.

Components of Physical Fitness

As noted in chapter 1, the three basic components of a physical fitness program are cardiovascular (aerobic) endurance, muscular strength, and flexibility. Build a basic conditioning program around these three elements and then include activity-related components (such as agility) or functional movements. Although your goal may relate primarily to one of these components, such as strength, a good program includes all three. Each has specific benefits related to your health and fitness and indirectly helps you with a variety of activities.

As you design a program to meet your needs, the goals you have set help you decide what to emphasize in your program. If you have a health-related goal such as improving your cardiovascular health (thereby decreasing your risk of cardiac disease), emphasize activities of a moderate intensity that last for at least 10 minutes. Such activities, however, do not have to be specifically exercise activities. I make a distinction between general health and physical fitness and place activities on a continuum, from those that meet basic health needs to those that improve fitness. Activities that improve physical fitness require a higher level of intensity and specificity. For health purposes, 30 minutes of activity accumulated throughout the day is adequate, whereas for fitness purposes one needs aerobic activity of longer duration per session. This book focuses on fitness, which provides more health benefits.

Before you construct your program, you should understand some underlying terms and principles. When I work with patients, my goal is that they take control of their own rehabilitation. If I only have them exercise under my supervision, telling them what to do without explaining the purpose of the activity, then I have not done my job properly. Usually such patients go home and do nothing. Then they probably develop problems again and need another visit to a health care professional that they might have avoided. Before discussing how to put together a program, then, I will explain a few important scientific concepts and exercise principles.

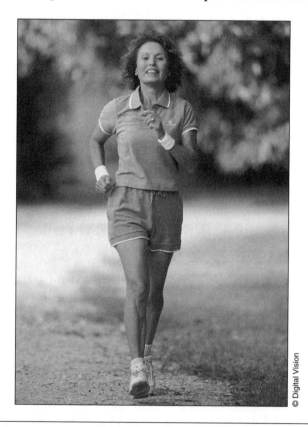

© Digital Vision

The type of exercise program you choose depends on your fitness goals and your personal needs; walking, for example, develops cardiovascular endurance.

Cardiovascular Endurance

Many terms are broadly synonymous with cardiovascular endurance, including aerobic fitness, aerobic capacity, and endurance. For my purpose, I emphasize the ability of the heart to deliver oxygen to the working muscles and their ability to use that oxygen. Many people think that physical activity and exercise are synonymous, but although exercise is a type of physical activity, not all physical activities are exercise (Whaley and Kaminisky 2001). For example, working in your yard is a physical activity and does have some health benefits, but it is not exercise. The best aerobic exercises are activities that raise your heart rate to a training level, last more than about five minutes, are repetitive in nature, and use a large muscle mass.

Some of the most common aerobic exercises are walking, jogging, swimming, and cycling. Exercise performed on indoor equipment can also be aerobic, if it is rhythmic in nature and uses a large muscle mass. Devices that simulate cross-country skiing, stair stepping, and rowing (along with many new devices on the market) can be used for aerobic exercise. Other activities, such as aerobics classes and tennis, do have some aerobic benefits. Because they usually involve only short bursts of activity, however, they do not produce the same degree of cardiovascular conditioning (although some of them may be appropriate for you). I address alternative exercise programs, especially group activities, in chapter 6 and give you pointers on what to look for in a class, if your goal is improved cardiovascular fitness.

Not only does aerobic exercise improve circulation to the muscles and joints, but the rhythmic nature of the activities also seems to help lubricate joints, thereby decreasing pain. Aerobic exercise is one of the easiest ways to reduce the stiffness associated with arthritis. An additional benefit is better maintenance of bone mass, which slowly starts decreasing after our 20s and can be a major health problem (Westby 2001; Minor et al. 1989).

Muscular Strength

Defined most simply as the ability to produce muscular force, muscular strength is often divided into muscular strength and muscular endurance. Muscular endurance is the ability of a muscle to contract repeatedly or continuously (as when carrying a child), whereas pure strength is the amount of force produced for one contraction (as when standing up from a chair). Most of us need a combination of the two—muscular endurance for posture muscles, and muscular strength in the trunk, legs, and arms for lifting.

Many people start losing strength as they age or become inactive, although the loss is not irreversible (Rogers and Evans 1993). In addition, women lose more strength than men do, especially from the upper body (perhaps because they may be less active when they are younger). Muscular strength allows you to perform many tasks at home and at work and, more important, helps to reduce the stress on joints. Hurley and Hagberg (1998) state, ". . . muscular strength is a major determinant of an older person's ability to maintain an active, high-quality lifestyle. . . ."

A top bodybuilder in the 70s age group reported that she started lifting weights because she had problems lifting grocery bags and doing other household chores. Amazingly, she did not start lifting weights until she was in her 70s. She is now in her 80s and looks great. I show her picture to my students and ask them to guess her age; they are always a couple of decades low.

Nervous system control of a muscle and the condition of the muscle itself combine to produce the muscular control and strength that various activities require. In fact, much of the initial gain from strength training is a fine-tuning of the amount of neural input that is required to contract a muscle. An example is the process by which toddlers learn to stand. Through repeated attempts, their movements become smoother and they are able to stand for longer periods. The amount of muscle contraction necessary for the activity has been refined, as has the strength in the muscle itself.

When there is pain around a joint such as your knee, the nervous system can also inhibit muscle contraction. Many patients have told me about a knee buckling unexpectedly, usually secondary to pain. After starting a strengthening routine, they have less pain and fewer problems with their knees giving way. Postsurgery joint replacement patients also illustrate the inhibition of muscle contraction because of pain. I see many patients the day after surgery who cannot lift their legs off the bed, even though they had no problem doing so before the surgery. As the pain around the surgical site decreases and they practice movements, these patients are able to lift the surgical leg again, even though there is no real change in strength. Most strengthening programs produce both neural and muscular changes that improve one's muscular control and strength (Sale 1988).

Flexibility

Flexibility is a broad term that includes several concepts. At its simplest, flexibility is the ability of a joint to move through its range of motion—for example, touching the shoulder with the hand. A motion becomes more complex when it uses several joints and muscles in combination. Touching one's toes, for instance, requires flexibility in the hamstrings, hips, and low back muscles.

A primary concern of many arthritis patients is being able to perform motions that require several joints to move in several directions. Golfers must be able to rotate and extend the shoulders at the same time that they flex and rotate the trunk, if they wish to produce adequate motion for a swing. Even everyday activities such as showering require the ability to move both shoulders in combination to wash the hair or back.

Joint flexibility is often lost with arthritis, but this loss is usually due to restricting one's movements because of pain. Increasing activities may delay the loss of flexibility and maintain function in a joint (Chapman, DeVries, and Swezey 1972). If one does not move a joint through its complete range of motion, one eventually loses a portion of its total motion. I worked with a lady who came to me because she could not raise her arm above her shoulder and as a result could not fix her hair properly. I found that she had lost shoulder strength from not using the arm and had also lost motion in her shoulder joint. Because her shoulder hurt when she raised her arm, she had quit raising it. With therapy, she was able to regain most of her range of motion and the ability to fix her own hair. If she had kept using the joint, perhaps modifying the activity to reduce the pain, she would not have required prolonged therapy to restore lost motion. The old axiom of "use it or lose it" rings true for one's physical abilities.

Related to flexibility is the concept of stiffness, one of the hallmarks of arthritis. Stiffness can be described as the "feeling of discomfort or restriction of movement after a period of inactivity" (Nichols 2001). In other words, it feels as if your joints and surrounding muscles need oiling. Stiffness, however, is not a true loss of a joint's range of motion. What often happens is that as a person starts to feel stiff, he moves less and may eventually lose full range of motion. One most often has this feeling after being in the same position for a prolonged time, such as sitting at the movies. Flexibility activities involve slow, gentle movement that decreases the sensation of stiffness and allows you to get moving again. I usually tell people to get up and move around every hour or so, moving all joints; just a little movement significantly decreases their sense of stiffness. See the sidebar for other ideas for reducing stiffness.

Conquering Stiffness

Stiffness is almost inevitable for arthritis patients, but here are some ways to gain the upper hand over it:

▷ Get up and move every hour.

▷ Take warm showers.

▷ Soak hands in warm water, performing range of motion activities in the water.

▷ Use a hot pack on the back (for no longer than 20 minutes) if there is no swelling.

▷ Apply creams or topical analgesics, which may reduce the pain associated with stiffness.

▷ Use a neoprene wrap to help keep a joint warm and decrease stiffness.

Functional Fitness

Although not included as one of the primary components of a fitness program, functional fitness may actually be the force driving your decision to start a fitness program. A person's underlying strength, endurance, and flexibility determine his ability to do typical household chores or work-related activities. Studies show that arthritis affects these underlying components as well as a person's ability to perform daily functions.

As you proceed with your program, you should notice an improved ability to complete everyday tasks. In fact, you may even have set goals specifically related to a task you were struggling with. Sometimes it is useful not only to have a traditional exercise-training program, but also to include specific functional activities within the program. For example, the patient who had lost her shoulder range of motion could not brush her own hair. As part of her home program, she practiced reaching toward her head while holding a brush. She had to work on this reach several times a day, while looking in the mirror. This exercise enabled her to see progress in her ability to carry out a daily function and complemented the rest of her rehabilitation program.

Warm-Up and Cool-Down

Including warm-ups and cool-downs in an exercise program becomes especially crucial as people age, recover from injuries, engage in vigorous activities, and confront health problems such as heart disease. The warm-up is a short period of gentle activity before the exercise session that prepares the muscles, joints, and other systems for exercise, while the cool-down period helps one slow down after exercise. Just as you personalize your exercise program, so you can adjust the warm-up and cool-down to meet your personal needs and suit your activities.

If you are very stiff you may want to do some gentle rhythmic motion, starting with small movements and increasing the range of the movements as you loosen up. For example, before playing tennis you can warm up your shoulders with pendulum swings. Begin with your arms at your sides and gently start swinging them with small pendulum motions, gradually increasing the range of the swing. A common variation of this warm-up is to hold your arms out from your sides at shoulder height. Make small circles, again increasing the size of the circle with each rotation. You can do other variations, but the objective is always controlled movement with a slowly increasing range of motion.

After this simple warm-up activity, add a slight stretch for your shoulders by reaching toward the sky, bringing your hands together over your head, and bending slightly to each side. These easy motions decrease stiffness and increase the blood flow to your shoulders, preparing them for strenuous activity. To complete your warm-up, you should perform a similar routine using your trunk, hips, and legs. Tennis is a whole-body activity, so your whole body needs to be prepared. Finally, you can practice some shots, simulating the moves you will use in a game and integrating more total body motion.

After an injury, the muscle or joint is stiffer and needs a gentler activity before exercise. In general, your warm-up should be proportional to the activity you will be doing. The more intense the activity, the longer the warm-up. If you are planning a 20-minute walk at a moderate intensity, you may not need much in the way of warm-up. Before walking, you may just stretch your calf muscles and then start out slowly, gradually increasing your pace. The gradual start can serve as part of your warm-up. Before a round of tennis, on the other hand, you must take more time to prepare all of the joints and muscles that are involved in playing the game. To warm up for a vigorous activity, I suggest gentle loosening-up exercises along with some movements to get your heart rate up. In addition to stretching your shoulders, jog around the court and do some trunk, hip, and leg stretches. When you were in your teens or 20s you might not have needed much warm-up, but warm-up becomes more important as you age, or if you are not fit.

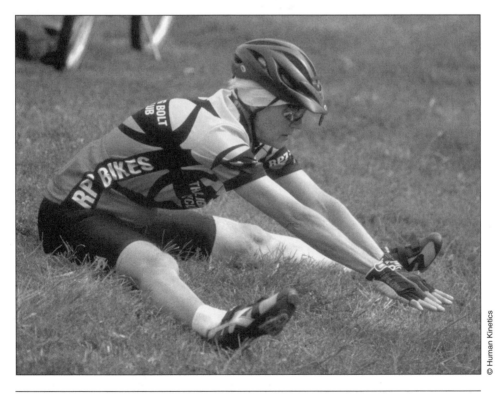

© Human Kinetics

Proper warm-up and cool-down are vitally important to maintaining your body's flexibility and preventing injury.

The cool-down, like the warm-up, must suit the activity you are doing and is more important for people who are not fit or who are older. If the activity is strenuous, the cool-down should be longer even if you are fit. This cool-down period is an important time for your body to get rid of some of the metabolic by-products that have been produced in your muscles (such as lactic acid). It also allows your other body systems to come back toward resting levels. Both warming up and cooling down decrease the possibility that a serious problem, cardiac arrhythmia, will occur (McArdle, Katch, and Katch 2000).

While in graduate school, I learned the hard way that if I did not cool down properly, I would pay later. After a difficult race I immediately sat on the ground, doing nothing. A short time later, I needed help to get up and was stiff for several days. One cannot prevent all soreness and stiffness, but I firmly believe that a good warm-up and cool-down routine can reduce their severity. Cooling down is now a regular part of my routine and if I was stiff before I exercised, then I lengthen my cool-down. I incorporate my stretching program into the cool-down, which seems to decrease stiffness the following day (especially if I have done a hard workout).

Exercise Principles

Several principles of exercise explain why and how variations in your program affect your body's response:

1. Overload
2. Progression
3. Specificity
4. Reversibility

Understanding each of these principles helps you personalize your program. Later I will discuss guidelines for applying these principles in relation to each component of fitness.

Overload

The first principle of training is that you must overload a system to stimulate a training response. If one can do something without much effort, then the body does not need to adapt. As a task becomes more difficult, the body adapts according to the stress that is put on it. It takes little muscular effort for a person to lift a pen, so the muscles do not adapt physiologically. If one is not used to lifting heavy objects, however, it takes greater muscular effort to lift several books. This overload to the muscular system stimulates changes in strength as one repeats it. A person may be able to walk down the block and back without too much stress. If one increases the speed or length of the walk, the effort overloads the system slightly and, with repetition, strengthens the cardiovascular system. One can accomplish an overload through several means, the most common being to increase the intensity, duration, and frequency of the activity. As I discuss each type of exercise in the chapters that follow, I provide guidelines for progressing that type of exercise (although you must apply these guidelines cautiously and personalize them for your body).

Note that overload operates along a continuum. A certain amount produces a good training response, while too much overload increases the chance of injury. If you have not been active and have decided to start a cardiovascular exercise program, I recommend starting with walking. For an initial program walk several times a day at a comfortable pace, for only 5 to 10 minutes at a time. As this amount is more than you were doing previously, it overloads the system—but not so much that you develop an injury. One gentleman that I know decided to start walking after a layoff due to injury, only to have to take more time off because he started with an hour walk and had severe knee pain the next day. The idea that if a little is good for you, a lot is better does not necessarily hold true for exercise.

Progression

One of the common causes of injury is improper progression—increasing the overload too quickly. The basic concept is that in order to allow the body to adapt properly to a training program, one must progress the program slowly and appropriately. This principle applies even to the starting level of a program. If your current activity level is low, do not suddenly increase it to a vigorous level. Often the body can temporarily adjust to an excessive overload, but the chance of incurring an injury is much greater. Most of us can think of a time when we did a lot of work around the house and could barely move the next day. We overloaded the muscles beyond what they were ready to handle.

An equally important aspect of this principle, however, is that in order to create an overload, one must progress the program. If a person walks every day for 20 minutes at the same speed, she will reach a point when she is maintaining her cardiovascular fitness but not advancing it. This state may not be bad if she has reached the level she desires, but to improve further she must progress her program. I have had many patients complain that they were not getting stronger, even though they were doing their home exercise programs. Upon analyzing their programs, I found that they were doing the same exercises they were doing when they first left rehabilitation—they had reached a plateau. The principle of progression says that if a person wants to improve, the amount of work must change. For many of these patients the change was as simple as increasing the amount of resistance they were using.

Several factors determine the rate of progression, including age, previous experience, past injuries, the type of exercise involved, and current health. Most initial adaptations to exercise are neural changes; the body becomes more efficient at recruiting only the amount of muscle required and initializing the various physiological systems needed during exercise. As a person ages, the body relies even more on neural adaptations for some forms of exercise. In addition, one's ability to adapt slows down with increased age or health problems. Young children master new skills quickly, but older adults sometimes struggle to learn them. On the other hand, if a person has done an activity before, his neural system adapts more readily (thus the old adage about never forgetting how to ride a bike).

The process of healing also slows with aging, so one must progress more slowly after an injury to allow the tissues time to heal properly. Arthritis is similar to injuries in that it affects not only the joints but also the surrounding muscles, so the progression of activity must be slower. In some instances, one may even need to decrease exercise intensity slightly after an illness or arthritic flare-up and then build back up from this lower level. After he had a severe pulmonary infection, I had my father start by walking the length of a few houses, two or three times a day, even though he had been used to walking several miles before his illness. Because of his prior activity level he was able to progress steadily; he added a house or two each day and was back to his normal mileage within a month or two.

Specificity

Specificity means that changes in your body are specific to the type and focus of training. If one performs strengthening exercises for the arms, one gains strength in the arms. Such an exercise may have some benefit for the entire body, but strength training the arms has limited aerobic benefits, since the primary purpose of the exercise is to provide muscular resistance. The concept of specificity also applies within a class of exercise, such as cardiovascular exercises. Someone who walks regularly may quickly be out of breath when swimming a lap at the pool. Walking moves the legs and arms in a particular way, with the legs doing most of the work. Swimming motions are entirely different; one primarily uses the arms. Any cardiovascular exercise has some crossover benefits; your choice of training activity may be affected by what your problematic joints can tolerate.

I briefly addressed specificity in chapter 1, when I discussed measuring your baseline. I suggested that you select a cardiovascular measure that would reflect the activity you are doing or plan to do. If you choose a different activity from the one that you used for a baseline measure, you may not see as much improvement as is actually occurring. Functional activities are quite specific, which is why they are good components of a training program. That very attribute, however, also limits their benefits. Remember the lady with the shoulder problem who practiced lifting her hand to her head as part of her rehabilitation. If she had done only that, with no other strengthening and flexibility exercises, she probably would not have been able to do other activities such as putting objects away in an overhead cupboard. Specificity, then, is one of the reasons you need a balanced program with cardiovascular, strength, and flexibility exercises.

Reversibility

Reversibility is the "use it or lose it" concept. The reversibility principle states that if we stop exercising, we will lose the physical capabilities that we are no longer using. This sequence occurs with many individuals when they are having problems with arthritis—they slowly decrease their activities and as a result lose flexibility, strength, and endurance. However, the principle works both ways; a person can reverse the effects of a sedentary lifestyle. With regular activity the body adapts and gains strength, flexibility, and endurance, regardless of the age at which one starts exercising.

This principle also applies to short periods of inactivity, such as being ill. If you have to stop exercising due to illness, you rapidly start to lose muscle mass and strength. As soon as you start exercising again, however, you can reverse the loss. As noted in the section on progression, you will need to decrease your exercise workload slightly upon resumption of your program. The longer you are not exercising, the more you will need to adjust your start-up level. Complete bed rest used to be the standard after surgeries and during illnesses, but we now recognize that complete rest is often not the best for healing. The rapid changes that occur in the body during bed rest may slow down healing. One of my jobs as a physical therapist is to help people get up and start moving, even the day after surgery. The changes are reversible, and the shorter the down time, the more rapid the recovery.

Ways to Stimulate a Training Response

Intensity, duration, and frequency are the three primary ways of overloading your systems. When you decide on your program, set the initial level for each exercise using a combination of these three.

Intensity

Intensity refers broadly to the amount of effort you put into an activity—whether it is fairly easy or fairly difficult for you to complete the task. The greater the intensity, the greater the training response (body adaptations such as getting stronger), at least to a point. The intensity of cardiovascular exercise determines how hard the heart has to work. The higher your heart rate, the more intense the activity, and we can therefore use our heart rate as a way of monitoring intensity of a cardiovascular activity.

The intensity of a strength activity, on the other hand, is related to how much force is required to move some type of resistance. As the amount of resistance increases, so do the amount of force one must exert and the resultant physiological response. Intensity, like overload, works on a continuum. At the lowest intensity an exercise does not elicit a training response, while at the highest intensity the chance of injury increases, as does the stress on bodily systems.

For example, your heart rate increases when you stand, but the increase is usually so minor that it does not stimulate a training response. If you suddenly jump up out of your chair and sprint to the door, however, your heart rate will probably rise to near maximal levels. Not only could you not keep going at a sprint pace, but you could also injure a muscle or sustain a more serious injury. Optimal training intensities tend to range from moderate to high intensity, and you must balance your workouts with appropriate recovery periods during which your body can make the necessary physiological adaptations.

Duration

Increasing the duration of an activity is the second way to overload the systems. The effect of increasing duration is easiest to demonstrate in cardiovascular activities. Most people can walk the length of a house without noticing fatigue or breathlessness. As one increases the length of the walk, however, the muscles need more oxygen and the heart must work harder, even when one walks at an even pace.

Strength training uses duration in two different ways—increasing the amount or time one holds a muscle contraction or, more commonly, increasing the number of contractions. Isometric contractions (ones in which you hold a position) may be timed. An example is the use of wall sits to strengthen your legs. You may start by holding a wall sit position for 30 seconds, gradually increasing the duration to 60 seconds. I do not usually recommend strength training by using a lot of long isometric contractions, because this method can have a negative effect on blood pressure. Though not normally thought of as a means of increasing duration, increasing the number of repetitions for a given movement also boosts the overload to the muscular system. Usually as the number of repetitions goes up, the amount of resistance (intensity) goes down, and the result is more improvement in muscular endurance. In general, 8 to 10 repetitions of a strength movement improve both muscular strength and endurance.

Frequency

Any workout may overload the system, but in order to bring about a training response one must continue to overload body systems on a regular basis. Many people do something once that is an overload, such as moving heavy objects in the house. Unfortunately, such an extreme overload to the muscles often results in soreness the next day and not in long-term changes. If you want to increase your strength, you have to overload the muscles on a more regular basis. Each of the three components of exercise—cardiovascular endurance, muscular strength, and flexibility—responds to slightly different frequencies of training.

Cardiovascular Requirements

To stimulate improvements in the cardiovascular system you must engage in aerobic exercise at least 3 times per week. You can increase the frequency overload by increasing the number of times per week. You can also increase the number of times per day that you exercise, although this is more commonly a way to reach the optimal duration of cardiovascular exercise when you cannot perform one continuous bout. For example, if you are just starting an exercise program, you can cycle 2 times per day, with each session lasting 5 to 10 minutes. You can also begin the frequency per week at the minimal 3 days, gradually increasing it to as much as 5 days per week.

Strength Requirements

The frequency recommended for strength training is a minimum of 2 times per week, although recent studies have demonstrated significant changes in strength with only 1 day per week (I will discuss different strength training options later). A frequency of more than 3 times per week is unnecessary and may set you up for injuries. Some of you have already had replacement surgeries or injuries that required rehabilitation. If so, a therapist may have instructed you to do your exercises 3 times per day. Such a "strength" program is only possible because you are not subjecting your muscles to a large resistance; these rehabilitation programs are designed to retrain the neural control of movement and build muscular endurance, not to increase strength. The gentleman who could not lift his leg off the bed after knee replacement surgery was told to do single leg lifts (among other exercises), increasing to 30 repetitions, 3 times per day. After the surgical site healed and he was back to normal activities, I put him on a resistance-training program, with a frequency of 2 times per week.

Flexibility Requirements

To improve flexibility one must do range of motion and stretching activities daily. Regular, gentle movement or stretching is essential for loosening stiff joints or movements. Once you have reached your flexibility goal, a maintenance program usually requires less frequency, although you probably ought to keep your flexibility program at the same level. Some muscles, such as the hamstrings, tend to tighten more easily and always need regular stretching. Tight muscles increase your feeling of stiffness and can alter the way that you move, putting unwanted stress on your joints. I have found that stretching for a few minutes a day greatly reduces stiffness in my legs and helps alleviate my low back pain.

Putting It All Together

Now that I have covered some basic principles and components of exercise, I will introduce some examples of entire programs. These examples show only overviews of the programs. The next few chapters address specific ways to set up or modify each separate component. Notice that a person does not have to do each type of activity every day; I will discuss specific guidelines later.

Using Your Goals and Baseline Tests

Before you start planning your exercise program, pull together your goals and baseline information. I find that it is easier to make a plan when I have all the preliminary information in one form (see the form on page 45). When you have each specific objective outlined, it is easier to decide which area to focus on or what type of activities you need.

Another way to keep track of this information is with an exercise log. You do not need anything fancy; you can make your own using a simple spiral notebook. Keeping a log serves two purposes—it helps you keep track of progress toward goals with objective information, and it actually helps you stick to your program. Daily training information to keep track of includes date, type of activity, duration, intensity, and symptoms. The method of recording intensity can be simple (such as labeling the activity hard or easy) or more precise (such as recording your heart rate). The symptoms record may help you spot an increase in problems related to a specific activity, leading to modifications of your program. You should at least have a log for your strength-training program to let you know the appropriate settings and resistance for each lift. If you do not want a complex log, keep track of your workouts in some manner. My mother likes to record her workouts on her calendar, because it gives her good visual reinforcement to stick with her program.

Matching Exercise Components to Goals

For someone who is just starting and whose goal is basic fitness, I suggest placing the greatest emphasis on cardiovascular exercise (as that has the greatest health benefit) while also building some strength and flexibility

SAMPLE OF INITIAL EXERCISE INFORMATION

Date: February 10, 2001   **Weight:** 145 lbs.

Current activity level: Walking 3 times per week for 15 minutes at a time

Goals:
1. Increase the amount of time I can walk without fatigue.
2. Decrease stiffness in my hands and shoulders so I can get objects out of the upper cupboards.
3. Decrease pain in my knees.
4. Lose 5 pounds.

Baseline assessment:

Walking test: 16:42 time, estimated $\dot{V}O_2$max of 32 (average fitness category)

Abdominal strength: 15 sit-ups (poor category)

Trunk and shoulder strength: 4 push-ups (very poor category)

Sit-and-reach test: 18.5 inches (fair category)

Shoulder flexibility: fair category

Objectives from baseline tests:
1. Decrease time for walking test, improving to good fitness category.
2. Improve in both strength categories to fair.
3. Improve flexibility to good category.

---

work into the program (see table 2.1). Note that the warm-up is relatively short on the days when the activity is walking and longer on the days when it is strength training. As you will see in the next chapter, people can even begin with several short sessions, such as a 5-minute walk in the morning, at lunch, and in the evening, if they are unable to tolerate longer walks at the beginning.

Next, look at a program for a golfer whose goals are to walk nine holes of golf without fatigue and to increase his flexibility for playing golf. Because he is already somewhat active (plays some golf), he can start with a slightly more intense level of aerobic activity. In order to follow the principle of specificity, the program sticks to walking. To address the person's flexibility goal, the program increases the flexibility component; it uses some activities specific to golf as well as some general stretches, but emphasizes stretching the shoulders and trunk. See table 2.2.

What if you are already doing regular aerobic activity, but are having problems with pain, stiffness, and loss of motion in your legs? I would suggest these program goals: (1) maintain cardiovascular conditioning, (2) decrease resting pain to 3 on a 10-point scale, and (3) increase hip and

Table 2.1   Beginning Program for Fitness

Days	Warm-up	Workout	Cool-down
Monday, Wednesday, Friday, Saturday	2-5 minutes: gentle movement of stiff areas and lower extremities	Walking: start with 15 minutes, comfortable pace (40% heart rate reserve (HRR), chapter 3)	5-10 minutes: stretching of lower extremities, trunk exercises
Tuesday, Thursday	10 minutes: 5 min cycling or walking; 5 min gentle movement of stiff areas, focusing on shoulders and lower extremities	Strengthening: 15 minutes—basic strength program (chapter 4): leg presses, hamstring curls, bench presses, biceps curls, lat pull-downs, hip extensions, hip abductions, rows	5-10 minutes: stretching of areas that have been stressed

Table 2.2   Sample Program for a Golfer

Days	Warm-up	Workout	Cool-down
Monday-Saturday	5 minutes: gentle movement of lower extremities (ankle circles, calf stretches, partial squats)	20 minutes walking: 5 min easy pace at beginning, 15 min brisk pace (60-70% HRR)	15 minutes: 2-5 min easy pace walking; flexibility program, emphasizing trunk and upper extremities
Sunday	5-10 minutes: gentle shoulder and trunk movement	Golf	

knee range of motion (flexion and extension). Remember that strengthening muscles around a joint decreases pain. Therefore, you would design a flexibility program to improve your range of motion, and a strengthening program to build up muscular support around the lower-extremity joints, as exemplified in table 2.3.

When you put together your program, you need to make sure that it fits your needs. We have all seen suggested training programs (usually more elaborate than the previous examples) in magazines or articles. Such programs, however, may not match your goals, abilities, or restrictions. If you have a very busy schedule, you may not have the time or desire for

Table 2.3   Sample Program to Increase Lower Extremity Range of Motion and Strength

Days	Warm-up	Workout	Cool-down
Monday, Wednesday, Friday	10 minutes: cycling with low resistance; gentle range of motion for lower extremity	Strengthening: 15 minutes—basic lower extremity program (chapter 4): leg presses, hamstring curls, hip abduction and adduction, hip internal and external rotation; start with high reps, low resistance until pain decreases	10 minutes: 5 min cycling; 5 min lower extremity stretching (hamstrings, calves, quadriceps, and hip muscles—chapter 5)
Tuesday, Thursday, Saturday	5-10 minutes: range of motion for lower extremity (chapter 5)	Your normal aerobic activity	10 minutes: lower extremity stretching (chapter 5)

a complex program. That is why it is helpful to understand some of the basic principles and guidelines of exercise; you can design or modify a program to fit your own needs and achieve your personal goals.

I saw a patient many years ago who had started a flexibility program that she found in an article on low back pain, which she was experiencing. She did not know how to personalize the program to her needs, unfortunately, and was seeking help because the program as outlined took more than an hour to complete. With a large, busy family, she was not able to stick with the program, and her back pain had increased. She did not need many of the recommended stretches—the program had stretches for every area of the body—and besides, the recommendations were not in line with underlying research. The program instructed her to hold each stretch for 1 minute, with 10 repetitions of each stretch. As you will see in the chapter on flexibility, this procedure does not follow basic guidelines for stretching. After altering her home program to a few stretches and adding some simple strengthening exercises, she was able to complete her daily program in 15 minutes; this program met her need for a short, simple workout and relieved her low back pain.

I have introduced the basic components and principles of exercise in this chapter and have discussed the need for you to individualize your program. You need to know more specifics about each one, however, in order to tailor your exercise plan effectively. The next chapter focuses on cardiovascular fitness—what it is, what activities stimulate it, and how to design the cardiovascular component of your program.

ACTION PLAN:
DESIGNING A PROGRAM

☐ Know the core components of fitness:

- Cardiovascular endurance
- Muscular strength
- Flexibility
- Functional fitness
- Warm-up and cool-down

☐ Understand exercise principles:

- Overload
- Progression
- Specificity
- Reversibility

☐ Understand the concepts of intensity, duration, and frequency.

☐ Compile your goals and baseline information and use them to personalize a program for your needs.

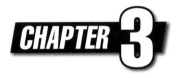

CHAPTER 3

ADDING AEROBIC ACTIVITY

You may have seen articles and health reports noting the importance of aerobic activity. Stiffness and pain from arthritis may have led you to think that it was your greatest health concern or that you could not participate in aerobic activities. Perhaps you are exercising but realize that you need to adjust your program—to add other components or modify existing activities—because of your arthritis. I remind patients that the number one cause of mortality for people over the age of 30 is heart disease, not arthritis. Furthermore, regular activity and exercise usually decrease arthritis symptoms and, contrary to popular belief, do not speed up deterioration in the involved joints (Panush and Brown 1987).

Benefits of Aerobic Activity

Aerobic activities are those that use oxygen to help produce energy in the active muscles. The heart, lungs, and circulatory system work together to get oxygen to the cells and to clear the byproducts of metabolism from the muscles. When a person is involved in physical activity on a regular basis, the cardiovascular system and the muscles involved in the activity reap the benefits of improved circulation. Regular aerobic exercise helps the circulatory and muscular systems become healthier and more efficient.

Not all activity is aerobic. The body can produce energy for a brief period (such as during a sprint) without the immediate use of oxygen. To be aerobic, an activity must last more than a few minutes and be performed at a sustainable intensity. Rhythmic exercises are excellent for bringing aerobic systems into play. They work the same muscles repeatedly, so that circulation does not have to switch from one area of the body to another. Exercises that fulfill these requirements include walking, jogging or running, swimming, and cycling. The aerobic classes do have some aerobic benefits but, because of the varied movements, the benefits are of a combined type—some muscular conditioning and flexibility on top of limited cardiovascular improvement. The cardiovascular gains, however, are not as great as those attained through the rhythmic exercises just mentioned.

Aerobic exercise benefits more than just your heart. Low-impact aerobic exercise does not exacerbate arthritis pain. Combined with strengthening and stretching, it improves fitness, decreases depression and pain, and (over the long term) improves function. Since several studies have found that the aerobic capacity of individuals with arthritis is lower than that of individuals the same age without arthritis, this aspect of fitness deserves attention (Ekblom et al. 1974; Beals et al. 1985; Minor et al. 1989). Health benefits accrue when a person simply transitions from inactivity to moderate physical activity (Whaley and Kaminisky 2001; Pate et al. 1995). As physical activity increases (in quantity or quality), the risk of cardiovascular disease decreases.

Some articles distinguish between aerobic activity and aerobic exercise—exercise being a more focused, intense activity. For example, mowing your lawn is an activity that yields some aerobic benefit, but not as much as taking a brisk 30-minute walk produces. Although I use the term

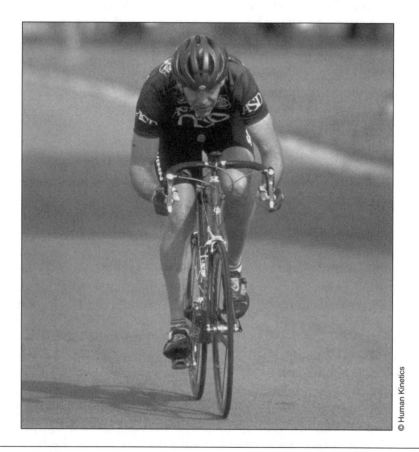

© Human Kinetics

Cycling as aerobic exercise is proven to have benefits for arthritis patients, and it also allows you to get outside and see new places.

aerobic activity throughout this book, I am referring to aerobic exercise. The health benefits of aerobic exercise include decreased risk of cardiac and other chronic diseases, normalized blood pressure, controlled body weight, decreased blood sugar and lipids, and decreased stiffness and pain from arthritis. Before identifying the basic requirements of an aerobic program, we must again examine the goals of the program, since they will help you decide on the appropriate level of each requirement within your exercise plan.

Basic Requirements of Aerobic Exercise

All of the fitness components need to meet minimum levels of overload in order to stimulate an adaptive response. Cardiovascular exercises are those that make the heart and lungs work harder than normal. Although the heart and lungs work more as soon as you transition from rest to any activity (such as getting out of a chair and walking to the kitchen) such increases are normally so mild that they will not cause improvements in the cardiovascular system. The amount of overload must be enough over resting level to challenge the system, but not so much over that the body cannot adjust.

Intensity

Our cells, muscular as well as other, have the ability to work both without oxygen (anaerobically) and with oxygen (aerobically). In order to work aerobically, the intensity of the activity must be such that the circulatory system can deliver oxygenated blood to the working cells. If the activity is too intense, the amount of oxygen may not be enough for the cells to work completely in the aerobic system; they must meet part of the energy needs without oxygen. This process produces lactic acid, and the body cannot sustain this level of activity for very long.

I often refer to track events to demonstrate the difference between the two systems. A quarter-miler (who runs one lap of the track) runs at a much greater speed than a miler, but he cannot maintain that speed for very long. If a miler starts a race at the same speed as the quarter-miler, he must slow down during the second lap—otherwise he cannot continue. You can demonstrate this phenomenon yourself. Raise your arms to shoulder level (don't do this if you have shoulder problems) and start making small, rapid circles. Not only will your heart and breathing rates rise rapidly, but you will also start to feel a burning sensation in your shoulder muscles and you will eventually stop. If you want to keep going, you must decrease the intensity by slowing down the speed of the circles and lowering your arms. Your breathing and heart rate went up to try to increase the amount of oxygen to the working muscles; when you slowed down the activity your circulatory system was able to meet the needs of those muscles, and you could keep going.

The rise in heart rate is directly related to the intensity of an activity—the more intense the activity, the higher the heart rate, at least up to a point. You have a resting heart rate (which is like your baseline) and a maximal heart rate (which is the highest your heart rate can go). Maximal heart rate is related to age, and the most common formula for estimating maximal heart rate is to subtract one's age in years from 220. Because of the linear relationship between heart rate and exercise intensity, you can assess your exercise intensity by monitoring your heart rate.

The American College of Sports Medicine (ACSM) has developed exercise guidelines for the healthy adult based on numerous studies (Pollock et al. 1998; ACSM 2000). The recommended intensity for aerobic exercise, in order to get a training response, is at 50 to 85 percent of a person's heart rate reserve (HRR). Heart rate reserve is a method of adjusting one's estimated maximal heart rate using one's resting heart rate. The sidebar shows the formula for finding your heart rate reserve, called the Karvonen formula, and includes an example of estimating intensity. The heart rate to aim for during exercise is usually called the target heart rate. I recommend using the Karvonen formula because it gives you a more appropriate heart rate if you have a resting heart rate that is very low or very high.

Estimating Training Heart Rate Using the Karvonen Formula

Maximal HR (MHR) = 220 – age

Training HR (THR) = [(MHR – resting HR) × intensity] + resting HR

Example: Age = 50 years, resting HR = 80, desired intensity = 65 percent

MHR = 220 – 50 = 170

THR = [(170 – 80) × .65] + 80

THR = 138.5 bpm

Assessing Your Intensity

Heart rate is easiest to take using the radial pulse, as described in chapter 1 (see figure 1.1 on page 13). Take your pulse on the wrist using the index and middle finger of the opposite hand, applying gentle pressure. If you use your thumb, which has its own pulse, you will get a false rate. Practice by taking a 30-second pulse, but during exercise you will take a 10-second pulse immediately after completing the activity. Multiply the 10-second count by 6 to calculate your heart rate in beats per minute (bpm). Your heart rate decreases rapidly once you stop exercising, so a 30-second heart rate underestimates your actual exercise heart rate.

Table 3.1 gives 10-second counts for target heart rates so that you can memorize your target 10-second count. Since taking a radial pulse has

Table 3.1 Ten-Second Heart Rate Counts With Minute Equivalents

10-second count	Beats per minute	10-second count	Beats per minute
10	60	21	126
11	66	22	132
12	72	23	138
13	78	24	144
14	84	25	150
15	90	26	156
16	96	27	162
17	102	28	168
18	108	29	174
19	114	30	180
20	120		

some room for error and using a 10-second count can exaggerate this error, aim for the target 10-second count, plus or minus 2 beats. For example, the training heart rate identified in the sidebar is 139; the target 10-second count would then be approximately 22 to 24, or 132 to 144 bpm. Trying to reach an exact heart rate is impractical and frustrating, while aiming for a target heart rate range is much easier.

If you take medication that alters your heart rate response, have problems taking your pulse, or want a simpler approach to estimating intensity, you can use what is called your RPE—rating of perceived exertion (Robertson and Noble 1997). For this method, estimate your exercise intensity on a scale ranging from 6 to 20 points. The scale is related to your heart rate; if you multiply the scale value by 10, it equals your heart rate. An RPE of 14 (exercising somewhat hard) corresponds to a target heart rate of 140. Therefore, if I determine that my target heart rate for an intensity of 60 percent is 140, my corresponding RPE should be 14. Rating of perceived exertion is not as accurate as measuring your heart rate, but with practice you will be able to estimate your response to exercise. If you are not on medications that affect your heart rate, you should take an exercise pulse at least once and relate it to your perception of work. Otherwise, use the descriptions of the levels to help you determine if you are at the correct exercise intensity: 13 to 14 = somewhat hard, 15 to 16 = hard, 17 to 18 = very hard, and 19 to 20 = very, very hard.

Setting Your Intensity

Determining the initial intensity for your program is based on several factors, including age, current activity level, exercise precautions identified by your physician, and the type and severity of your arthritis. Most clinicians agree that the older and less fit you are, the lower the initial intensity should be. You are more likely to stick with a program if you minimize the intensity at the start, such as beginning at 40 percent of HRR, which is lower than the range of intensity normally suggested (ACSM 2000). Starting with a light workload decreases the chance of soreness and injury and limits the aggravation to your arthritis. Later in the chapter, I address the major types of aerobic exercise and give examples of initial intensities for different types of people.

When in doubt regarding your own program, err on the side of caution. It is much better to start out at a level that might be too easy for you and then progress the intensity than to start out at too high an intensity. By starting out easy you can develop the habit of exercising and reduce your chance of injury. See table 3.2 for recommendations on intensity level based on a person's current level of activity.

Table 3.2 Recommended Initial Intensity Based on Current Activity Level

Current activity level	Intensity
Sedentary (less than 2 days/week, mild activity)	55-65%
Mildly active (2-3 days/week, mild to moderate activity)	65-75%
Active (3-5 days/week, moderate to vigorous activity)	75-85%

A simple way of telling if you are at the right level during exercise (without stopping to take a pulse during the session) is the talk test. At the lowest intensity you should be able to carry on a conversation with your partner while exercising. At a moderate intensity you will probably be able to say a sentence or two but will not want to talk constantly, since you will feel breathless. At a vigorous level of aerobic exercise, you will be able to answer a question or make a short statement but will not want to talk much more than that. Remember—if your working muscles get a heavy, burning sensation, you are working too hard. The burning sensation generally signifies the production of lactic acid, a by-product of metabolism when the muscle is not getting enough oxygen (a process that I described earlier).

As you advance, you may want to vary intensity by using different training methods. Although most of the programs outlined here focus on continuous work, with more challenging programs you might include two other techniques: interval and fartlek. Interval exercise involves alternating periods of exercise and rest, or even alternating periods of intensity. The ratio of rest to the exercise interval determines which metabolic system you will use. The shorter the rest period, the more aerobic the session. The rest intervals are not always complete rest, but relative rest—meaning you slow down your pace but keep going. Fartlek, which means "speed play" is a technique developed in Sweden. It involves a continuous session, with varying levels of intensity. For example, the first few minutes of the workout can be easy; then comes a short burst of intense speed, followed by a moderate pace for a longer period. This variation in intensity continues throughout, but the intervals are not necessarily equal. Both of these techniques are good ways to vary your exercise session and stimulate additional systems, such as those used for speed.

Duration

As noted previously, it takes several minutes of continuous activity to start to use the aerobic systems effectively. The longer you maintain the activity, the greater the percentage of energy derived from the aerobic system. The guidelines from the American College of Sports Medicine identify a goal of 20 to 60 minutes of continuous, aerobic activity. Once again, your initial duration must be based on current level of activity, age, and other health parameters. Because of your arthritis you may need to start with 5-minute bouts of exercise, resting in between (Minor 1996). You then slowly lengthen your session toward the recommended duration. If you have been mildly active you might increase your initial duration to 15 minutes; someone who has been very active can easily start out with 20 to 30 minutes.

These initial durations may seem extremely short, but you can compensate for the brief duration by increasing the frequency of your sessions, such as engaging in two to three bouts of exercise throughout the day. Starting with too long a duration, as with too great an intensity, may lead to soreness and potential injury. As one ages it takes slightly longer to adapt to physical stressors and one is at greater risk for certain types of overuse injuries. Your joints, tendons, and muscles need time to adapt to the new stresses you are placing on them.

Some of you may need or want to stay with shorter bouts. Sometimes work schedules make longer exercise sessions difficult to fit in, whereas two 15-minute exercise bouts work into a schedule more easily. Some people tell me that a shorter session does not aggravate their arthritis, but when they try to increase their exercise time, they start having more pain. You must find what duration of exercise works for you, both in terms of your schedule and your arthritis. In the long run, it is much better to exercise regularly than to stop exercising because you could not do the "ideal" program.

Staying Hydrated

Preventing dehydration is extremely important, especially when you're exercising. Follow these tips to keep yourself hydrated.

▷ Drink plenty of water and juices throughout the day.

▷ At least 1 hour before a longer exercise session, drink 1 to 2 glasses of water or an electrolyte replacement drink (try a small portion to make sure it does not upset your stomach).

▷ During longer sessions, especially when it is hot, drink small amounts every 15 to 30 minutes.

▷ Immediately after exercising, replenish the fluids that you have lost by drinking water, juice, or an electrolyte replacement (with greater sweat losses, an electrolyte replacement is preferable). The amount of fluid loss is related to temperature, intensity of activity, duration of activity, and your body weight.

▷ Alcohol and caffeine are dehydrating substances—avoid them or at least decrease your consumption if you will be exercising later.

Frequency

How often you exercise each week is a crucial factor in your response to the program. For health benefits you should (ideally) do some sort of activity every day. The Centers for Disease Control and Prevention (CDCP) and ACSM guidelines for cardiovascular health suggest activities (not necessarily exercise) on "most, preferably all, days of the week" (Pate et al. 1995). The recommendations for cardiovascular fitness are similar, with a minimum of 3 to 5 days of aerobic exercise per week (ACSM 1998; 2000). The potential for injuries increases as the frequency and duration of exercise increases (especially over 5 days per week). One way to decrease the chance of overuse injuries is to do another activity, such as cycling, once or twice a week, or to reduce the intensity to a mild level. The health benefits of a regular fitness program far outweigh the risk of injury with a properly designed program.

As I mentioned in the section on duration, you may need to divide your exercise sessions into two separate periods per day. This increase in frequency during the day is only appropriate when your aerobic exercise session is shorter than desired. The total daily time for your sessions should not normally exceed the recommended guideline of 20 to 60 minutes. Although there are no criteria for what are considered maximal time limits, I suggest that 60 minutes be your maximum. Beyond this you may be at risk of overuse due to the effects of arthritis—better safe than sorry.

Aerobic Activities

As noted, activities that are continuous, rhythmic, and use larger muscle groups stimulate the cardiovascular system optimally. The most common of these exercises are walking, running, cycling, and swimming. I will discuss some of the benefits that have been identified for each activity and make suggestions for using that mode of exercise.

Walking

Walking is an excellent activity and a functional one as well; we all have to walk to get around. A walking program can improve endurance, aerobic capacity, and walk time while decreasing pain and depression in people with arthritis (Minor et al. 1989; Minor 1991). You can do it daily as long as you vary the intensity and follow some basic advice.

As with any activity, equipment can increase or decrease your chance of injuries. The most important pieces of equipment for walking are socks and shoes. If you have arthritis in your lower extremities, chances are that your biomechanics are altered and your walking gait is not ideal. Proper shoes can help improve limb alignment and gait, resulting in a more even stride and less stress to your arthritic joints. If you are like me, you may look at the cost of a good pair of walking shoes and think that you don't need them that much. However, poor shoes may actually worsen your gait and heighten the stress on your arthritic joints, thus increasing the long-term damage. Your physician may even decide that you need orthotics or special shoes, which may be covered under your health insurance if the physician prescribes them.

Do I Need Special Walking Shoes?

Although walking shoes are not required, I do recommend them because they are designed for the biomechanics of the activity. A good shoe for walking will provide comfort, shock absorption, and support, especially through the arch. Make sure that you have plenty of room in the toe box and that the heel counter fits closely around the heel to prevent slipping. Shoes and other joint protection strategies are addressed in more detail in chapter 7. Socks may not seem important, but they do add cushioning and decrease potential friction. Make sure your socks are absorbent and fit properly. Check your shoes and socks regularly for wear, and replace them when needed. Worn-out shoes can lead to overuse injuries or increase the stress on your arthritic joints, causing increased pain.

What Type of Warm-Up Should I Do?

A warm-up for a walking program emphasizes gentle movements that use the entire body, such as reaching to the sky. It concentrates on the calves (heel cords), hamstrings, quadriceps, and hip muscles. Chapter 5 discusses the different types of stretching and range of motion exercises. For activities that do not call for rapid, ballistic motions, stretching before the activity does not appear to be as important for preventing injury as stretching after the activity. Nevertheless, the muscles and systems that will be stressed need to be warmed up. Active stretches, such as range of motion movements, get blood flowing to the muscles. Do 5 to 10 repetitions of each range of motion. If you are feeling stiff, add some short stretches. After a few warm-up moves, you can start with a slow walk and then gradually increase your speed until you have reached your target intensity. Remember, you should feel that you can maintain this speed (intensity) throughout your walk.

Where Should I Walk?

Walking surface is a concern with arthritis, because uneven surfaces place more stress on lower-extremity joints and increase the possibility of injury. Hills can be very difficult, especially if they are steep, and can cause increased pain in the involved joints. Walking down stairs or hills alters the biomechanics of movement and transmits more stress to the lower extremities. Start out on fairly even, flat terrain. You might add some gentle hills as you become stronger, but realize that steep hills may cause problems—regardless of your fitness level—if your joints are severely compromised.

Walking indoors at a mall or on an indoor track is a good alternative to walking outside on varied terrain, especially if the weather is poor. If you walk in a mall, adjust your intensity (particularly if it is crowded), and make sure to wear well-cushioned shoes. Walking on a treadmill is also a good option. Safety is a concern when walking on a motorized treadmill, so make sure you know how to get on and off of it safely. A good treadmill should have an emergency stop button, which can help prevent falls. I have found that walking on a treadmill can be very boring; music or a television can provide a distraction and make the session more enjoyable.

I am often asked about using some sort of stair-stepper as a form of walking exercise. This type of exercise is aerobic and can be beneficial; however, some people with arthritis have told me that it aggravates their knee or hip pain. Based on this feedback, I don't generally recommend it to arthritis patients. If you want to try a stepper, I suggest you start by setting it for a low resistance, a small step, and a short duration so that you can see how your joints react to this activity.

What Does a Walking Program Look Like?

Tables 3.3, 3.4, and 3.5 lay out walking programs for individuals with three different starting levels: previously sedentary with low fitness, mildly active with fair to moderate fitness, and currently active with good fitness. Possible progressions through a three-month time frame are shown for the first two examples, while shorter progressions are shown for the others.

Please remember that these are only examples and that you must tailor any program to suit your needs and abilities. One's health status and response to a program also determine how it progresses. For example, if you find that the initial workout length is quite easy, and if you are not sore, you may increase the duration from 5 minutes to 10 minutes for the second workout. As long as pain or stiffness does not increase, it is still a safe duration for early in your program. If you increase the duration and your knee swells up, however, back off to the workout's previous length and take steps to control the swelling. If you were not having any problems before this incident, review the previous few days' activities—you might find that something else is the culprit (such as walking on an uneven surface the day before).

Note that for the individual with low fitness in table 3.3, the initial intensity is lower than the ACSM guidelines; it is modified to accommodate arthritis and to help the person stick to the program. The intensity stays low for a few weeks and then slowly increases, as does the duration. Notice that the frequency starts at three times per day, which brings the total time toward the recommended minimum. The workout frequency can be decreased to twice a day as the sessions approach 15 minutes in length, then to once a day when they last about 20 minutes. From then on the person can slowly increase both intensity and duration.

A person who has been somewhat active and is at the fair to moderate fitness level (based on a preliminary fitness evaluation, if possible) can begin with longer walks at a higher intensity (see table 3.4). The intensity of the workout remains steady during the first month, but the duration increases. It is tempting to ratchet up speed and duration more rapidly, but arthritis patients are more likely to stick with a program if it progresses slowly and stays within comfort levels for their arthritis. It is often wise to increase duration without increasing speed until you get used to working out.

You may find that you are in better shape than you thought, or that your arthritis is not bothering you much. In this case, you might increase the intensity by 2 to 5 percent in the fourth week. If you were closer to the moderate level of fitness for your baseline test, you might start with a single bout of 20 minutes and then increase duration, intensity, or both.

An active individual who wishes to implement a regular training program or modify an existing one can start off at a higher level of intensity (see table 3.5). I would suggest putting some variations into this program to keep it interesting and challenging. Do what you prefer, however—some people like a consistent routine so that they do not have to check a log to see what to do. To vary the regimen you might include a hilly route or a longer walk two times per week (see week 1 in the table).

Table 3.3   Initial Walking Program for Individual With Poor to Fair Fitness

Month 1	Month 2	Month 3
WEEK 1		
Frequency: 3-5 days/week* Intensity: 40% of HRR Duration: 5 minutes, 3 times/day	Frequency: 5-7 days/week Intensity: 45% of HRR Duration: 15-20 minutes, 1 time/day	Frequency: 5-7 days/week Intensity: 50% of HRR Duration: 30 minutes, 1 time/day
WEEK 2		
Frequency: 3-5 days/week Intensity: 40% of HRR Duration: 6-7 minutes, 2-3 times/day	Frequency: 5-7 days/week Intensity: 45% of HRR Duration: 20-25 minutes, 1 time/day	Frequency: 5-7 days/week Intensity: 50% of HRR Duration: 30 minutes, 1 time/day
WEEK 3		
Frequency: 3-5 days/week Intensity: 42-43% of HRR Duration: 10 minutes, 2-3 times/day	Frequency: 5-7 days/week Intensity: 45-48% of HRR Duration: 25-30 minutes, 1 time/day	Frequency: 5-7 days/week Intensity: 55% of HRR Duration: 30 minutes, 1 time/day
WEEK 4		
Frequency: 3-5 days/week Intensity: 42-43% of HRR Duration: 12-14 minutes, 2 times/day	Frequency: 5-7 days/week Intensity: 47-48% of HRR Duration: 30 minutes, 1 time/day	Frequency: 5-7 days/week Intensity: 55% of HRR Duration: 30 minutes, 1 time/day

*Alternate days if only 3 days/week

As the program intensifies, the warm-up and cool-down gain in importance. Each should be lengthened, incorporating more range of motion exercises, more mild aerobic activity (such as marching in place), and more stretching—especially during the cool-down. Include strengthening work for your trunk and lower extremities, which guards against injuries and problems that can occur on hills or rough terrain. Many people take it for granted that if they have been walking regularly, their trunk and legs have acquired the strength they need. This assumption is not true. According to the principle of specificity that I discussed in chapter 2, strengthening occurs primarily through exercises that require you to produce more force. Walking builds endurance in your muscles, but not necessarily strength.

Table 3.4   Intermediate Walking Program for Individual With Fair to Moderate Fitness

Month 1	Month 2	Month 3
Week 1		
Frequency: 5 times/week Intensity: 55% of HRR Duration: 15 minutes, 2 times/day	Frequency: 5-7 times/week Intensity: 57-58% of HRR Duration: 25 minutes	Frequency: 5-7 times/week Intensity: 62-63% of HRR Duration: 30-35 minutes
Week 2		
Frequency: 5 times/week Intensity: 55% of HRR Duration: 17-18 minutes, 1 time/day; 10 minutes, 1 time/day	Frequency: 5-7 times/week Intensity: 57-58% of HRR Duration: 30 minutes	Frequency: 5-7 times/week Intensity: 62-63% of HRR Duration: 30-40 minutes
Week 3		
Frequency: 5 times/week Intensity: 55% of HRR Duration: 20 minutes, 1 time/ day; 10 minutes, 1 time/day	Frequency: 5-7 times/week Intensity: 60% of HRR Duration: 30 minutes	Frequency: 5-7 times/week Intensity: 65% of HRR Duration: 30-40 minutes
Week 4		
Frequency: 5 times/week Intensity: 55% of HRR Duration: 22-23 minutes	Frequency: 5-7 times/week Intensity: 60% of HRR Duration: 30-35 minutes	Frequency: 5-7 times/week Intensity: 65% of HRR Duration: 30-40 minutes

Chapter 4 addresses strength training and provides some ideas for training your trunk and legs. One gentleman with whom I worked walked regularly, often for several miles. He never did any strength training, however, and could not walk down stairs easily. After a simple home strengthening program, he could not only get up and down stairs more readily but also found that he could walk faster and with less pain.

Jogging or Running

Some misconceptions about jogging need to be addressed. Jogging or running is not for everyone with arthritis, but it has acquired a bad reputation among older people over the years, perhaps unjustly. When I was preparing to write this book, a professional colleague told me that he hoped I would not discourage people with arthritis from running. A runner

Table 3.5 Advanced Walking Program for Individual With Good to Excellent Fitness

	Week 1	Week 2	Week 3	Week 4
	Frequency: 5-7 times/week Intensity: 75% of HRR Duration: 30-45 minutes	Frequency: 5-7 times/week Intensity: 75-80% of HRR Duration: 30-45 minutes	Frequency: 5-7 times/week Intensity: 75-80% of HRR Duration: 30-45 minutes	Frequency: 5-7 times/week Intensity: 75-80% of HRR Duration: 35-50 minutes
Mon	30 minutes	30 minutes	35 minutes	30 minutes
Tues	35 minutes	35 minutes, 80% HRR	40 minutes	40 minutes, 80% HRR
Wed	30 minutes, hilly route	35 minutes, hilly route	40 minutes, hilly route	45 minutes, hilly route
Thur	30 minutes	40 minutes, easy	45 minutes, easy	35 minutes
Fri	35 minutes, hilly route	35 minutes, hilly route	30 minutes, hilly route, 80% HRR	40 minutes, hilly route, 80% HRR
Sat	45 minutes, easy*	45 minutes, easy	45 minutes, easy	50 minutes, easy

*Easy—decrease intensity by about 5-10%

himself, he had often been told that he should give up running because it would cause arthritis.

Some people suggest that running either leads to or worsens arthritis. Most of these theories are based on the fact that running does have a higher impact on the lower extremities than walking. While it is true that the impact on joints from running is considerably higher than from walking, there is little evidence that running by itself leads to arthritis. A few studies have examined the incidence of arthritis related to running, with findings on both sides. Those studies that noted an increased incidence of arthritis in runners found that high mileages and fast training paces appeared to raise slightly the risk of developing the disease. Some larger epidemiological studies have found previous joint injury, along with gender and obesity, to be the most predictive factors; they also concluded that running, jogging, and other strenuous physical activities did not increase the chance of developing arthritis (Morrow et al. 2002; Hootman 2002).

In fact, the relationship between the risk of developing arthritis and running appears to be a U-shaped curve. There is a slight increase in risk at high levels of running, but moderate levels may actually provide some protection—the other end of the curve shows an increased risk of arthritis from lack of activity. No evidence exists that individuals with arthritis who continue to run will accelerate their arthritis (Lane et al. 1987; Fries et al. 1994).

How Do I Get Started?

If you have not been running and are at a low aerobic fitness level, start with walking and see how you respond, progressing through a program to the vigorous level. In conjunction with the walking program, start strengthening your lower extremities. Then, if you want to run, begin by alternating walking with jogging.

If you were a runner in the past, you can start jogging at an easy pace for short periods, 15 to 20 minutes, as long as you have not gained much weight over the years and do not have significant lower-extremity arthritis. Extra weight is a primary risk factor for arthritis and, combined with a high-impact activity such as running, may put undue stress on your joints. If you are overweight, stick with walking or another low-impact activity until your weight is more appropriate for your height.

If you are already running, you do not have to stop simply because you have been diagnosed with arthritis. Often an increase in joint pain leads a person to consult a physician, who diagnoses the disease. Try decreasing your mileage temporarily, during which time you can implement a strengthening program and get your pain under control. Once the pain is under control, slowly increase your mileage back toward your desired level. You may find that you can continue running but need to keep your mileage lower than what you could maintain comfortably in the past. When I was in graduate school, I trained for marathons. Although I still run, I have found that my knee starts giving me problems with too much mileage. In order to keep running, you may need to compromise between what you want to do and what your body can withstand.

Do I Need Special Shoes?

Because of the harder impact of running, the shoes you wear and the surface you run on require careful attention. Chapter 7 makes some suggestions for running shoes. Make sure that your shoes provide adequate cushioning and foot control. Replace your shoes more frequently than you would for a walking program; do not try running in worn-out shoes.

Notice that I include strengthening in the suggestions for training, even though this section covers running. A key to success with my own program has been my strengthening regimen; it has greatly decreased my knee pain after jogs. Studies show that knee strength is lower in individuals with arthritis. Increased muscular strength helps to absorb the force of impact that running transmits through one's lower extremities.

What Does a Running Program Look Like?

Keep your mileage or run duration low unless you are aiming toward a competition (such as a 10K race). Running for 30 to 60 minutes per workout is more than adequate for fitness; also make sure to leave a day or two for rest. Varying the mileage or duration during the week is a common training technique that not only decreases boredom but also allows better recovery.

In the sample program for someone who is ready to start running (table 3.6), I recommend keeping to fairly flat terrain. Alternate walking and jogging, gradually decreasing the amount you walk. The example alternates 5-minute periods of walking and jogging during the first week, changing to 10-minute sections the next week. Even if your baseline fitness is good enough for you to start a jogging program and you have been doing some exercise, it is best to start slowly—allow your joints and muscles time to accommodate the higher impact of jogging. If you are impatient, however, start with short jogs, as I suggested previously.

If you are currently running and just want to modify your program, you have numerous options. The example in table 3.7 is only one suggestion. As with a walking program, a varied running program fights boredom, but you may find that time or location constraints dictate a mostly constant routine. You can still vary distance, type of terrain, and intensity, or experiment with techniques such as fartlek.

Cycling

Cycling is an excellent aerobic activity, especially if you want to decrease joint impact. I know several people who switch to cycling when their arthritis is acting up, as a way of exercising without pain. Most studies have dealt with stationary cycling, so you may get different results if you opt for an outdoor cycling program. The important consideration is that cycling, like other aerobic activities, has proven benefits for individuals with arthritis.

What Are the Best Cycling Settings?

Two factors in a cycling program can affect knee and hip pain during the activity: seat height and pedal resistance. Adjust the seat height so that your knee is almost completely extended when the pedal is at its lowest position (see figure 3.1 on page 67). This setting allows the greatest range of motion through your knees and hips and disperses the stresses. If you are built like my father (who is 6 feet, 4 inches tall), you may need to have your seat mount modified to allow for greater height; with outdoor cycles, look for a larger frame. Keep the pedal resistance at a low setting, which permits a higher turnover rate. You can set this up easily on a stationary cycle via the resistance control mechanism. When riding an outdoor cycle, utilize a wide range of gears and shift to an easier resistance with hills.

Table 3.6 Intermediate Jogging Program for Individual With Good Fitness Level

Month 1			
Week 1	**Week 2**	**Week 3**	**Week 4**
Frequency: 5-7 times/week Intensity: 65% of HRR Duration: 20-30 minutes, alternating 5 min jog, 5 min walk	Frequency: 5-7 times/week Intensity: 65% of HRR Duration: 20-30 minutes, alternating 10 min jog, 10 min walk	Frequency: 5-7 times/week Intensity: 65-70% of HRR Duration: 20-30 minutes, continuous jogging	Frequency: 5-7 times/week Intensity: 65-70% of HRR Duration: 20-40 minutes
Mon 20 minutes	20 minutes	20 minutes	20 minutes
Tues 25 minutes	25 minutes	25 minutes	30 minutes
Wed 30 minutes	30 minutes	30 minutes	40 minutes
Thur 20 minutes	20 minutes	20 minutes	30 minutes
Fri 25 minutes	25 minutes	25 minutes	20 minutes
Sat 30 minutes	30 minutes	30 minutes	40 minutes

Month 2			
Week 1	**Week 2**	**Week 3**	**Week 4**
Frequency: 5-7 times/week Intensity: 70-75% of HRR Duration: 20-40 minutes	Frequency: 5-7 times/week Intensity: 70-75% of HRR Duration: 30-50 minutes	Frequency: 5-7 times/week Intensity: 70-80% of HRR Duration: 30-60 minutes	Frequency: 5-7 times/week Intensity: 70-80% of HRR Duration: 30-60 minutes
Mon 30 minutes	40 minutes	40 minutes, hilly	40 minutes, hard
Tues 30 minutes	40 minutes, hilly	45 minutes	50 minutes
Wed 40 minutes	50 minutes	30 minutes, hard**	45 minutes, easy
Thur 20 minutes	30 minutes	50 minutes	30 minutes, hard, hilly
Fri 30 minutes	40 minutes, hilly	40 minutes	50 minutes, easy
Sat 40 minutes	50 minutes, easy*	60 minutes, easy	60 minutes

*Easy—decrease intensity by 5-10%

**Hard—increase intensity by 5-10%

Table 3.7   Advanced Running Program for Individual With Good to Excellent Fitness

	Week 1	Week 2	Week 3	Week 4
	Frequency: 5-7 times/week Intensity: 70-80% of HRR Duration: 30-45 minutes	Frequency: 5-7 times/week Intensity: 70-80% of HRR Duration: 30-50 minutes	Frequency: 5-7 times/week Intensity: 70-85% of HRR Duration: 30-60 minutes	Frequency: 5-7 times/week Intensity: 70-85% of HRR Duration: 30-60 minutes
Mon	30 minutes, hard**	30 minutes, fartlek	35 minutes, hard	40 minutes
Tues	40 minutes	45 minutes, hard	45 minutes, easy	50 minutes, hilly
Wed	45 minutes, fartlek	35 minutes, hilly	50 minutes, hilly	45 minutes, hard
Thur	40 minutes	50 minutes, easy	45 minutes, fartlek	30 minutes
Fri	35 minutes, hilly	35 minutes, hilly	30 minutes, hard, hilly	40 minutes, easy
Sat	45 minutes, easy*	50 minutes	60 minutes, easy	60 minutes

*Easy—decrease intensity by 5-10%

**Hard—increase intensity by 5-10%

The comfort of the seat also affects your ease during cycling. Many new types of seats are available, which are usually wider and have better padding than older bicycle seats. Try out the seats to see what is most comfortable for your body build. Lastly, bicycling (especially outdoors) can cause problems with your wrists. Find a bicycle on which you can modify hand positions and maintain a relatively upright posture. You may even want to put padding on the handlebar to decrease the discomfort in your wrists and hands.

One variation of the stationary cycle that you may consider using is the type in which the handlebars can move in synchrony with the pedals (for example, the Schwinn Aerodyne). These machines usually permit an upright posture and, because of the position of the handlebars, reduce the stress on your wrists. They also allow you to work your upper body throughout the exercise, which provides better conditioning, flexibility for the trunk and shoulders, and greater comfort. The American College of Sports Medicine has information, available over the Internet, on selecting a stationary cycle. This resource also is listed on page 181.

What Does a Cycling Program Look Like?

If you have not been active, especially with cycling, start out with no resistance during the warm-up period, and keep the resistance very low

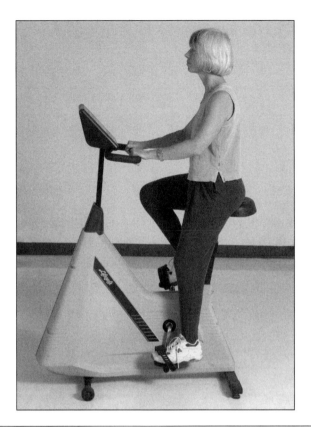

Figure 3.1 Proper position on a cycle.

for several weeks (see table 3.8). This strategy helps to reduce soreness in your thighs. If you are outdoors, keep to relatively flat areas for the first few weeks. Start with a low intensity, based on your lack of previous activity. Your cool-down can also be done with no resistance and a slower pedaling rate. Sitting may not be comfortable at first, so start with two to three shorter exercise periods per day (although the example shows a 15-minute session) until you adjust to the seat.

If you have been cycling already, you can begin at a slightly higher intensity, but start and end your warm-up with no resistance. Because the cycling motion is very different from that of walking, your muscles work differently; if you have been active but not with cycling, you must go through an adjustment period. Finally, if you are already cycling and have started having joint pain, you may need to modify your program. A neoprene sleeve for your knees may provide some pain relief, while still allowing you to cycle. As with other aerobic activities, strengthening may help improve muscle balance and decrease excessive stress around your joints. Tight muscles may also be contributing to the problem, so be sure to work on your flexibility. If you have been cycling and are looking for some variety, use different paces and durations, similar to fartlek, even during a ride (see the example in table 3.9 on page 69).

Table 3.8 Initial Cycling Program for Individual With Poor to Fair Fitness

Month 1	Month 2
Week 1	
Frequency: 3-5 days/week Intensity: 50% of HRR; 50-60 rpm Duration: 15 minutes	Frequency: 5-7 days/week Intensity: 60% of HRR; 55-65 rpm Duration: 30 minutes
Week 2	
Frequency: 3-5 days/week Intensity: 55% of HRR; 50-60 rpm Duration: 20-25 minutes	Frequency: 5-7 days/week Intensity: 60-65% of HRR; 55-65 rpm Duration: 30-35 minutes
Week 3	
Frequency: 3-5 days/week Intensity: 50% of HRR; 50-60 rpm Duration: 20-25 minutes	Frequency: 5-7 days/week Intensity: 55% of HRR; 55-65 rpm Duration: 35 minutes
Week 4	
Frequency: 3-5 days/week Intensity: 55-60% of HRR; 55-65 rpm Duration: 25-30 minutes	Frequency: 5-7 days/week Intensity: 55-60% of HRR; 55-65 rpm Duration: 40 minutes

For outside cyclists, I must put in a word about helmets. A helmet is a critical piece of safety equipment—do not ride without one. Like me, you probably never wore a helmet as a kid and find them hot and uncomfortable. However, head injuries from cycling accidents are a serious concern, and you will soon get used to wearing your helmet (if it helps, think of the example you are setting for young persons).

Swimming

When I was in college, an elderly gentleman with severe rheumatoid arthritis used to come to the pool every day at lunchtime and swim laps in the diving pool for the entire hour. I saw him do this for four years; he rarely missed a session. He told me that swimming was the only thing that kept him moving and decreased the pain. Swimming is not for everyone, but there are many who swear by it. If your arthritis involves your shoulders, you may find that swimming aggravates rather than relieves your pain. However, those patients with lower-extremity arthritis or multiple

Table 3.9 Advanced Cycling Program for Individual With Good to Excellent Fitness

	Week 1	Week 2	Week 3	Week 4
	Frequency: 5-7 days/week Intensity: 70-75% of HRR Duration: 30-45 minutes	Frequency: 5-7 days/week Intensity: 70-75% of HRR Duration: 30-50 minutes	Frequency: 5-7 days/week Intensity: 70-80% of HRR Duration: 30-60 minutes	Frequency: 5-7 days/week Intensity: 70-80% of HRR Duration: 30-60 minutes
Mon	30 minutes	30 minutes	40 minutes, hard	45 minutes
Tues	35 minutes, varied pace	45 minutes, varied pace	50 minutes	50 minutes, varied pace
Wed	40 minutes	40 minutes, hard	35 minutes, varied pace	60 minutes
Thur	30 minutes	45 minutes, easy	40 minutes, hard	35 minutes, hard
Fri	45 minutes, varied pace	30 minutes, hard	50 minutes, easy	45 minutes, easy
Sat	45 minutes	50 minutes, varied pace	60 minutes, varied pace	60 minutes, varied pace

joint involvements may find that the lack of impact afforded by swimming makes it a great exercise choice. Swimming has several benefits: decreased weight bearing due to the buoyancy of the water, increased relaxation and reduced stiffness (with the proper water temperature), and total body conditioning.

What Does a Swimming Program Look Like?

I suggest starting with an interval program, since few people can swim continuously for the recommended duration if they have not already been doing some swimming (table 3.10). The upper body tends to decondition more rapidly than the legs. Swimming is not a functional activity, whereas people do some walking every day even if they are not training. Set a baseline, just as you would with the other activities. You can do the test identified in chapter 2, or you can simply see how many laps you can swim without stopping. This number will then become your initial interval length; if you can swim four laps without stopping, then you will try for four laps each time, resting between intervals. I recommend varying your stroke, which not only decreases the amount of stress from specific motions, but also makes the exercise more interesting.

Table 3.10   Initial Swimming Program for Individual With Poor to Fair Fitness

Month 1	Month 2
Week 1	
Frequency: 3-5 days/week*	Frequency: 3-5 days/week
Intensity: 50% of HRR	Intensity: 60% of HRR
Duration: 20 minutes total; intervals (see description in text)	Duration: 30 minutes total (continuous, if possible)
Week 2	
Frequency: 3-5 days/week	Frequency: 3-5 days/week
Intensity: 55% of HRR	Intensity: 60% of HRR
Duration: 20 minutes total; intervals—increase each interval by one lap	Duration: 35 minutes total (continuous, if possible)
Week 3	
Frequency: 3-5 days/week	Frequency: 3-5 days/week
Intensity: 55% of HRR	Intensity: 65% of HRR
Duration: 25 minutes total; intervals—continue to increase each by one lap	Duration: 35-40 minutes total (continuous)
Week 4	
Frequency: 3-5 days/week	Frequency: 3-5 days/week
Intensity: 55% of HRR	Intensity: 65% of HRR
Duration: 30 minutes total; intervals—continue to increase each by one lap	Duration: 40 minutes total

*Alternate days if 3 days/week

If you are already doing some swimming, then you can start progressing up to the optimal 30 to 60 minutes of continuous activity. As you will see in the example in table 3.11, I make interval training part of the sessions, using longer intervals, to keep the program interesting. I also suggest alternating strokes during the intervals and including some kicking (with or without a kickboard) and pulling (using pull buoys to support your lower-body weight) in the routine. Diversifying your program decreases boredom and perhaps lowers the risk of overuse injuries caused by employing only one stroke.

Are There Any Special Considerations for a Swimming Program?

Heart rate is lowered when one is in the water and when one swims. One suggestion is to subtract 13 beats per minute from your predicted maximal

Table 3.11   Advanced Swimming Program for Individual With Good to Excellent Fitness

	Week 1	Week 2	Week 3	Week 4
	Frequency: 3-5 days/week	Frequency: 3-5 days/week	Frequency: 3-5 days/week	Frequency: 3-5 days/week
	Intensity: 65-75% of HRR	Intensity: 65-75% of HRR	Intensity: 70-80% of HRR	Intensity: 70-80% of HRR
	Duration: 30-45 minutes	Duration: 35-50 minutes	Duration: 40-60 minutes	Duration: 40-60 minutes
Mon	30 minutes continuous	45 minutes continuous	40 minutes continuous, hard	40 minutes continuous, hard
Tues	45 minutes: 20 continuous, 15 hard intervals	50 minutes: 25 continuous, 25 intervals	50 minutes: 30 continuous, 20 interval	55 minutes: 35 continuous, 20 interval
Wed	40 minutes continuous	35 minutes continuous	40 minutes continuous	45 minutes continuous
Thur	45 minutes: 25 continuous, 10 intervals	45 minutes: 30 continuous, 15 intervals	60 minutes: 35 continuous, 25 hard intervals	60 minutes: 40 continuous, 20 interval
Fri	30 minutes continuous, hard	50 minutes, easy	50 minutes continuous, easy	50 minutes continuous, easy

heart rate and then calculate your target heart rate (McArdle, Katch, and Katch 2000, p. 377). This modification will provide a more accurate heart rate for swimming. Another way to adjust for the altered heart rate is to use perceived exertion to monitor your training intensity.

Swimmers often have problems with shoulder pain, partly because of the imbalance in muscular pull that develops with swimming. The anterior muscles become strong and tight, pulling the shoulders into a forward, rounded position. To counteract this pull, include in your program strengthening exercises for scapular (involving the posterior shoulder muscles) stability and a stretching program for the anterior shoulder. The butterfly stroke is especially stressful to the shoulder joint, so use it sparingly, if at all. Using paddles can also lead to problems; they provide more resistance for the anterior shoulder muscles, which leads to even greater muscle imbalances. This tendency to imbalance is also why I suggest limiting a swimming program to five days per week (at the most).

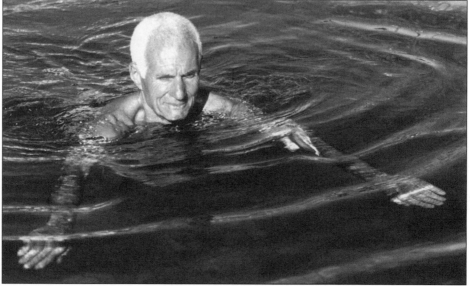

Swimming is an excellent, low-impact way to get aerobic exercise.

Personalizing Your Program

Personalizing your program means more than deciding if you will walk or swim, or if your program will start with the lowest intensity or a slightly higher one. It means adjusting the aerobic program that you believe you need to fit your lifestyle, available facilities, and personal needs or desires. I will provide some examples of personalized programs, but each person will have unique needs and wants.

An acquaintance personalized her program by combining a bicycling program with a swimming program. On Tuesday and Thursday, she does an evening lap swim at the local indoor pool. She bicycles to work on Monday, Wednesday, and Friday when the weather is decent, or does stationary cycling on evenings when cycling outdoors is not an option. She also likes to hike on weekends, adding a nice social activity while she gets some aerobic exercise.

My father likes to be flexible with his program, adjusting it to match the weather and his other activities. When he goes to the gym in the winter and early spring, he does stationary cycling for approximately 15 minutes and then walks on the treadmill for about the same time. After this aerobic exercise, he completes a weight program that we set up. He walks outside or cycles around the lake if the weather is decent. In the summer, he regularly walks 9 holes of golf and often takes additional walks. He prefers a home strengthening program when the weather is good, because it is easier to fit into his varied schedule.

If you are not in the habit of being active, I suggest that you write out your program and keep an exercise log. You can still personalize the routine to fit your schedule, but writing it out and using a log helps you stay on track. By analyzing your normal daily schedule, you can identify times during which you may have to adjust or vary your exercise routine. For example, if you work full time and have a standing meeting on Wednesday evenings, you can mark Wednesday as a rest day or perhaps opt for short walks in the morning and at lunch instead of exercising after work. I usually exercise after work, but on Fridays I used to have a standing lunchtime run with a friend. This gave me some social time as well as varying my routine. During the summer I adjust my schedule by not working out on Tuesday, which is my golf league day (I always walk the course).

Personalizing your program helps take it from a "have to" to a "want to" program and improves the chance of you sticking with it over the long run. It is also not a one-time adjustment. As you progress, you will not only modify your program's intensity and duration but also work in other exercise options. Perhaps you participate in a seasonal sport, such as golf, or you get involved with a group that exercises together as a social activity. In my town, a group of people meets every weekend at a local restaurant to walk, jog, or run. They come from all over town and are of varied fitness and talent. This weekly get-together is a fun social activity that reinforces their exercise programs.

The information and examples in this chapter all focus on cardiovascular exercise. The next component of exercise (identified in chapter 1) is strength. I have alluded to the importance of strength in everyday activities. In chapter 4, I will address the basic requirements of a strength-training regimen, types of strength-training programs, and some basic safety guidelines. Strength training is not just for young athletes; it is vital to everyone's exercise program.

ACTION PLAN:
ADDING AEROBIC ACTIVITY

- ☐ Measure your heart rate and determine your intensity level (the recommendation is 50 to 85 percent of heart rate reserve).
- ☐ Set your duration and frequency based on current level of activity, age, and health issues (recommendations are 20 to 60 minutes per day for at least 3 to 5 days a week).
- ☐ Choose an aerobic activity (or several): walking, running, cycling, swimming, or other.
- ☐ Use the sample programs and adjust them to your fitness level, schedule, and other needs.

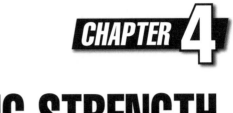

CHAPTER 4

BUILDING STRENGTH

Y ou may think that you do not need strength training or that it may cause more pain and stiffness, so why do it? As I have mentioned in previous chapters, strength training can actually provide several benefits. I started my father on a simple strengthening program several years ago, when he was putting off knee replacement surgery. He was able to delay having surgery for several years because of his regular exercise. When he finally had the surgery, he regained his functional strength relatively quickly. After finishing rehabilitation, he started on an intensive strength-training routine at a local facility. Now, not only is the leg with the replacement doing well, his other knee is hurting less.

Benefits of Strength Training

People with arthritis have found that strength training can reduce pain and improve strength and function, without worsening the arthritis. Knee arthritis patients who participated in a strength-training program three times per week reported significant gains in strength and in functions such as walking. They also found that simple tasks like putting on their socks were easier (Baker et al. 2001).

Strengthening exercises increase circulation to the exercising muscles and build lean muscle mass (thereby raising your metabolism). They can also extend the range of motion in some joints (Hurley and Hagberg 1998). Stronger muscles may absorb stress that is otherwise transmitted to the joint. Weakness in the lower extremities precedes and contributes to the pain and loss of function characteristic of arthritis (Wrightson and Malanga 2001). Finally, muscular strength is crucial if you are considering a joint replacement, since inadequate strength can slow down your recovery. I have worked with many patients who had to go to a rehabilitation facility after knee surgery because they were unable to get out of a chair without help; the other leg was too weak.

Basic Requirements of Strength Training

Remember that to stimulate adaptation in muscles, you must overload the muscular system. You can overload the muscular system by increasing the resistance against a movement or by increasing the frequency or duration of the resisted movement. You can choose from several methods of executing a resistance activity, each of which uses a different type of muscle contraction. As you age your body adapts to strength training primarily through neural changes; the muscles respond more efficiently and more completely when necessary.

Before you put together the specifics of a strength program, decide whether your goal is to improve muscular endurance, pure strength, or a combination of the two. Muscular endurance is the ability to maintain a contraction for a prolonged period, or to contract the muscle with some force repeatedly. An example of muscular endurance is carrying a bag of groceries into the house; usually you hold your arms in the same position the whole time. If you do not have the endurance necessary to complete the carry, you drop the bag. You use pure strength to lift an object one time with a short movement, as when you put a suitcase into the car. Most people need both of these types of strength, so go with a combination program if you are not sure what type of strength you need for your goals.

Improving Strength for Everyday Tasks

If you are frustrated with not being able to manage certain tasks or movements, here are some strength exercises that can alleviate these problems:

▷ Do you struggle to carry grocery bags into the house? Work on grip strength and do biceps curls, latissimus pull-downs, and rows.

▷ Do you suffer from low back pain during household chores? Strengthen your trunk with abdominal crunches, birddog moves, and plinth exercises. You also need thigh strength, because part of the pain may be from bending the back rather than the hips and knees. The leg press and hip extension exercises will strength these areas.

▷ Do you have difficulty getting into and out of a chair that has no arms? Thigh and leg strength is the key. Focus on the leg press and hip extension exercises.

▷ Do you have trouble with small chores around the house? Grip strength, often neglected, is a key requirement for accomplishing many household tasks comfortably.

If you are recovering from an injury or suffering from significant pain, you may need to begin with a program that emphasizes neuromuscular control. In such a regimen you use the same muscle again and again, overloading it primarily by repetitions. Therapists use this technique frequently; patients use lightweight rubber tubing for mild resistance, perform the same movement 15 or more times, and repeat the activity several times a day. This type of program is good for reducing pain and increasing motion in a joint before a regular strengthening program.

The ACSM guidelines for healthy adults recommend 2 days per week of resistance training (ACSM 2000; 2002). The guidelines suggest doing 8 to 10 exercises to work the major muscle groups. With regard to intensity, they recommend 8 to 12 repetitions per movement, using a moderate load. These guidelines sketch out an efficient program that will yield both muscular strength and endurance. If you desire a more advanced weight-training program, schedule a strength workout 3 days per week and do 3 sets of each exercise; this boosted level gives you greater benefits without overly stressing your arthritic joints. If you decide on a home exercise regimen, work out at least 3 days per week and add some functional strength activities into your daily routine.

Intensity

The intensity you use will depend, as mentioned, on the strength gains you desire and the goals you have set. Think of intensity as a continuum that ranges from no resistance to high resistance. The most common method of determining intensity for a resistance-training program is to discover your 1-, 6-, or 10-lift maximum for each movement. You then set intensity at a percentage of that lift.

Most systems identify a different intensity for each set within a 3-set regimen. This technique works well if you plan to use a gym or fitness center that has varied apparatus and someone who can help you determine your baseline for each movement. Another technique for determining starting resistance levels is based on body weight (Kisner and Colby 2002). The initial lifts are a percentage of body weight: for example, bench press = 30 percent of body weight; leg extension = 20 percent of body weight; leg flexion = 10 to 15 percent of body weight; and leg press = 50 percent of body weight. Otherwise, an easy option is to estimate what you can lift for a movement and then try it. If ten repetitions are extremely easy, then increase the weight the next time; if you cannot complete ten repetitions, decrease the weight.

For a general strengthening program, resistance will then be moderate to high, approximately 80% of maximum. Less resistance combined with a higher number of repetitions (15 to 20) will result in better muscular endurance. With arthritis, one of the most important factors determining the amount of resistance is your comfort level. Resistance training is not supposed to be overly easy, but if you start having more painful symptoms with your arthritis, back the resistance down. Most people tell me they have fewer problems with a low-resistance (about 50 percent) program that uses moderate repetitions (1 set of 10 to 15 reps). I usually initiate strength training with this type of program so that we can see how their arthritis responds.

If you plan to exercise at home, design a program that uses your own body weight, handheld weights, or simple resistance devices such as rubber tubing. You determine the intensity for such activities by the number of repetitions you can complete with full body weight or with a given resistance. If you cannot use your total body weight at first (as in a full push-up), you can start with a position that reduces the amount of weight you have to move, simulating a percentage of a maximum lift. For example, if you can do only one push-up on the ground, start with a standing push-up against a wall (see figure 4.1). This position works the same muscles but reduces the resistance. As you get stronger, you can eventually move to the ground to do your push-ups. Home exercise programs are usually less intense, but you can still gain valuable strength benefits with a properly designed regimen (Baker et al. 2001).

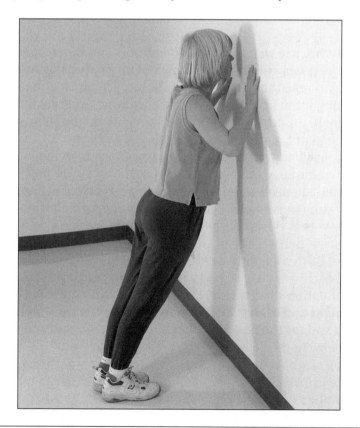

Figure 4.1   Wall push-up.

Progression

When and how much to increase resistance is always a concern when one is strength training. Numerous weight-training systems have been developed, but the most specific in terms of knowing when and how much to progress resistance is the Daily Adjustable Progressive Resistance Exercise (DAPRE) system developed by K. L. Knight (1979). This system is most helpful for those doing a formal resistance program that uses machines or free weights. A 6RM base (see chapter 1) is used to determine your workloads; use the following intensities and repetitions:

Set 1 = 10 repetitions at 1/2 of your 6RM

Set 2 = 6 repetitions at 3/4 of your 6RM

Set 3 = As many repetitions as possible at your full 6RM

Set 4 = As many repetitions as possible at adjusted load

Set the amount of these four loads. Then adjust your workout loads based on how many repetitions you are able to perform during set three. If you can perform only 2 or fewer reps during set three, decrease the load by 5 to 10 lbs. If you can do 3 to 4 reps, leave the resistance as it is. Increase the resistance by 5 to 10 lbs when you can perform 5 to 6 reps; by 5 to 15 when you can do 7 to 10 reps; and if you do 11 or more repetitions, increase the load by 10 to 20 pounds.

As you can see, this type of program can become complex, so I only recommend this approach if you are extremely serious about your resistance-training program and are looking for considerable improvements in strength. Pay attention to practicing proper biomechanics and keep close track of your symptoms with this intensive program.

A simpler method for determining progression uses your ability to increase the number of repetitions you do in a set. You know that it is time to increase the resistance or repetitions when you can do the exercise without strain—that is, when you feel you could easily do more. Increase your repetitions per set to 15. Once you can do 15 reps, increase the weight the next session by 5 to 10 pounds, and decrease the number of repetitions back to 8. If you cannot complete 8 repetitions at the new level, then you need to decrease the amount of resistance.

The most common mistake I see with people's programs is that they have not progressed the resistance. One gentleman, however, sometimes has me tearing my hair out; he increases resistance very rapidly, ignoring the concept of slow progression. He has sometimes increased a resistance exercise by two weight levels and more than doubled the number of repetitions from one session to the next. I definitely do not recommend this technique.

Even if you are using body weight or other types of resistance, such as rubber tubing, remember that intensity needs to be advanced in order to achieve greater strength. If you keep the resistance at the same level, with the same repetitions and frequency as when you started, you will plateau. When using rubber tubing, increase the resistance by switching to the next thickness. Most elastic resistance systems use a color coding scheme to denote the amount of resistance and have a reference to tell you which colors represent more difficult resistance.

For body weight activities, such as push-ups, increasing the resistance becomes challenging. Earlier I gave an example for push-ups—starting against a wall for low resistance and eventually progressing to the floor for high resistance. You can even alter the resistance in the floor position; doing a modified push-up with your knees on the ground reduces the amount you have to lift. If you use your feet as the lower contact point, the amount of body weight increases. You can progress the program as usual by raising the number of repetitions and sets, or if you really want a challenge, you can do the push-ups on a reverse incline. At home you can create an incline by laying face down in front of stairs and putting your feet on the bottom step to do the push-ups.

Frequency

The goals of your strengthening program determine the frequency of training. If you aim to improve your strength, traditional guidelines recommend three days per week, but newer guidelines suggest two days per week of resistance training. Two days yield satisfactory improvements in strength; you can realize greater strength gains with more days per week, but the added benefits are minimal. Even one day of strength training will improve your strength, although I recommend at least two days a week. Schedule a day of rest in between workouts to achieve optimal results. Competitive lifters and body builders train more frequently, but they alternate between lower body and upper body each day.

If you are starting a program for pain reduction or for rehabilitation (high reps, low resistance), do it five days per week. Therapeutic programs for such goals often call for patients to perform the activity two to three times per day; resistance is minimal, and the idea is to overload the muscle through frequency. A modified exercise-dosing scheme recommends that a person complete over 45 repetitions per set—doing 6 to 12 sets spread throughout the day—when the purpose is to reduce swelling and pain (Holten 1993). As pain or swelling subsides, the resistance goes up and the number of repetitions goes down; the frequency decreases to once per day.

Immediately after my father's knee surgery, he started on a simple program that included two strengthening exercises for his legs. He had to do these at least three times a day, working up to 30 repetitions per session. Once the surgical site healed, he added resistance in the form of rubber tubing to one of the exercises and performed it only once per day, with fewer repetitions. Eventually he progressed the other exercise (leg lifts) by adding cuff weights to his ankle and reducing both repetitions and daily frequency. When he finally started a program at the gym, he did this heavier training only two times per week, although he was encouraged to continue leg lifts at home on the other days.

Once you build up a moderate to high resistance, remember to include a day of rest between training sessions. You can still do some exercises daily, however, because the resistance usually stays at a mild to moderate level. These activities include low back stabilization exercises and some of the body weight activities that emphasize muscular endurance. See table 4.1 for guidelines.

Table 4.1 Resistance-Training Continuum Based on Training Goals

	Rehab/pain	Endurance and strength	Strength
Intensity	0-40%	40-60%	>85%
Reps	>20	12-20	<6
Sets	Multiple	3	3
Frequency	3 + times a day	2-3 times a week	2-3 times a week

Variations in Resistance Training

Two factors to consider when setting up a strength-training program are the type of muscle contraction you will use for an exercise and the kind of biomechanics to move the involved joints. The type of muscle contraction determines the potential tension developed within the muscle, its response to training, and possible soreness after workouts. Similarly, if your movement is dictated by a fixed path, such as with a weight machine, there may be a different response than if you move a resistance freely.

Type of Muscle Contraction

Three basic types of muscle contraction result from different movements—concentric, eccentric and isometric contractions. Both the concentric and eccentric contractions occur when you move a joint through a range, while the isometric contraction involves no movement. A concentric contraction is one that shortens the muscle. The eccentric contraction, often used when controlling the release of a movement, lengthens the muscle. You can easily see these types of muscular contractions when you perform biceps curls. As you lift the weight toward your shoulder, the biceps shortens concentrically, and when you return your arm to the starting position, releasing the move toward the ground, the biceps works eccentrically. You would perform the biceps curl against an immovable object to create an isometric contraction.

Many rehabilitation experts recommend using isometric resistance if your joint is inflamed, since the joint does not move. Both isotonic (moving) and isometric strengthening routines are effective for individuals with arthritis (Wrightson and Malanga 2001). While isometric routines do improve strength, they are not as effective as resistance programs that use motion. The strengthening benefit from an isometric exercise is primarily for the angle at which the resistance activity is performed, so it is often necessary to do several contractions at different joint angles. Because you are not moving the joint, an isometric exercise does not help you maintain total joint range of motion. Also, an isometric contraction actually reduces blood flow to the muscle, which causes blood pressure to rise.

If a joint is highly inflamed, you can perform brief isometric contractions, with repetitions (Lieberson 1984). This technique limits the blood pressure increase, while still giving the strength benefits. If your joint is not inflamed, I highly recommend doing your resistance moves through as much of the joint's range of motion as possible. In this way, you can maintain or even extend that range while reaping the benefits of increased strength.

Open Chain Versus Closed Chain Exercise

In addition to different types of muscle contraction, you can use two basic types of movement to elicit those contractions. Each has pros and cons, and you may need to analyze an activity to decide if you want to include it in your program. The names of these types of movement, open chain and closed chain, come from the science of biomechanics. They refer to whether or not the extremity is fixed at the distal end during an exercise, meaning whether the hand or foot stays in contact with either a stable surface or a piece of equipment that moves in a predetermined way. An open chain activity is one in which the extremity can move in any direction, because it is not attached at the end. For example, if you raise one of your feet off the ground, you can move that leg in any direction or sequence of movements. A closed chain activity, on the other hand, fixes the distal end of the extremity either to the ground or to a device that has a predetermined motion. When you keep your feet on the ground while you bend or straighten one joint, the other joints move in a predictable, set manner.

Open chain exercises do a good job of targeting one set of muscles for strengthening, but they increase the forces transmitted to the involved joint. Closed chain activities transmit less force to the joint (although they too can be stressful) and often are more functional movements. Another benefit is that when you perform closed chain exercises, you often strengthen several muscle groups.

Because of the increased stress on joints, keep open chain activities to a minimum. Exercises such as biceps curls are simple and usually do not cause too many problems. On the other hand, knee extension exercises that use an open chain motion produce a lot of stress to the knee and will probably increase your pain. If you opt for an open chain activity, keep the resistance lower around an arthritic joint. For example, you might do a knee extension in an open chain manner using rubber tubing, but keep away from knee extension machines. If you want to use a machine, the leg press is a better option; it is a closed chain activity and you can usually modify your position to further decrease the stress to your knees.

Home Versus Fitness Facility Program

I am often asked whether a client should join a gym. It depends on that individual's needs and personality and on the gym's accessibility, among other factors. Many people join health clubs each year and quit going to them within a few weeks. Before joining a health club, I suggest you answer a few questions:

1. Do you like to exercise with other people around?
2. Is the health club easily accessible? (Consider both its distance from your house and its hours of operation.)
3. Does the equipment suit your needs? Is it adjustable, and does the weight go low enough for you? (I have never heard of a patient who complained because the weight would not go high enough.)
4. How crowded is the facility during the hours when you plan to exercise?
5. Is there someone qualified to supervise a program for an individual with special needs such as yours?

Some of the better health clubs allow a trial membership, which lets you find out whether you will truly enjoy working out in that facility. After his preliminary rehabilitation program after knee surgery, my father went to a local health club that offered short-term (about 3 months) memberships. He discovered that there were special hours for seniors only, which were less crowded and during which a nurse with specialized rehabilitation training was available. Many health clubs that are associated with hospitals have special classes and equipment for individuals with arthritis. The variety of equipment available at most health facilities is a positive factor, and allows you greater creativity in designing your program. For some people, having paid a membership fee can be an added incentive to help them stick with a program.

What if you wish to improve strength but work out at home? You can devise an effective resistance-training program using your body weight, small handheld or cuff weights, or rubber tubing. As I noted earlier, you can reduce the resistance for body weight exercises by using a support or modifying the position. For example, an effective exercise for increasing quadriceps (front thigh muscle) strength is a squat; however, traditional squats can increase the stress to the knee joint. A modification that reduces the stress to the knee and helps to support your body weight is doing a wall squat. With your back to a wall, take two to three steps away from the wall and then put your back against the wall, lowering your body slightly. The angle of your bent knees should not go below 90 degrees. With the wall supporting you, you can hold this position for 30 to 60 seconds, which you probably could not do without the wall support or modification to the knee position (see figure 4.2).

Another way to modify this exercise is to put a large ball between you and the wall. The ball allows you to glide up and down, making it possible to perform repetitions of the exercise rather than a prolonged hold (make sure that you are stable if you do this sort of modification).

Employing rubber tubing or small handheld weights offers a way to build resistance while giving greater variety to your home program. Exercise tubing is available in several thicknesses; you can start with lightweight elastic and gradually progress the resistance, just as with weights. Advantages to tubing are its low cost and its portability—you can take it

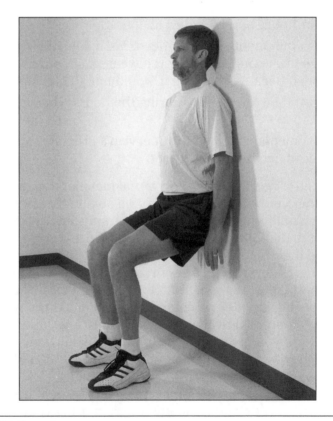

Figure 4.2 Wall squat.

anywhere. Many therapists use elastic tubing for rehabilitation programs because they can give it to patients to take home. One potential problem with tubing is that it wears out with repeated use and can then break, especially if you perform your exercises vigorously.

You can set up an effective home program with minimal financial output by selecting some cuff weights and a few dumbbells. Some of the new brands of equipment have adjustable weights, often using water or sand to fill the weight. However, you may find that you are only able to progress to a certain level, after which you are unable to increase the resistance without additional equipment. Obvious benefits of a home program are the reduced cost, lack of a crowd, and no need to travel.

Guidelines for a Safe and Effective Program

Following several basic guidelines will help make your program safer and more effective.

1. Start with exercises that work the major muscle groups, which include the trunk (chest, abdomen, and back), shoulders, hips, legs, and arms (ACSM 2000).

2. Include a warm-up and cool-down with each resistance session. A warm-up should have some aerobic activity, as well as gentle stretching.

3. Perform all exercises in a controlled manner, with proper technique. If you are not sure of a technique, seek help. If you have to use your entire body or a ballistic movement to move the weight, then the weight is too much—reduce it.

4. Do not hold your breath. Breathe out slowly while lifting and inhale as you release the weight (see section on the Valsalva maneuver).

5. Exercise both the front and back (both sides) of a joint to produce muscular balance around it. For example, work both the hamstrings and the quadriceps.

6. Use full range of motion for a joint, when possible. An exception to this guideline is performing squats; squats past 90 degrees increase the stress to the knee joint, with no added benefit.

7. Monitor your response. Decrease a load if there is increased joint pain, or discontinue it if there is new pain. Monitor your blood pressure if you have preexisting health problems.

8. Make necessary modifications, such as in the range of an activity, to accommodate your arthritis; use splints or gloves to decrease injury potential to a joint. Gloves may be especially helpful in decreasing the discomfort in your hands during lifting and may help you keep a better grip.

Recommended Exercises

You can develop a balanced strength-training program with a few basic exercises. Work opposing muscle groups in order to develop balance around major joints, and use muscle groups from the upper and lower extremities as well as from the trunk. Proper positioning and control are crucial during resistance training. Keep your spine in a neutral position, without excessive arching or forward bending. When you must bend for exercises such as reverse flys, bend from the hips. During standing upper body exercises, keep your hips and knees slightly bent.

Upper Body Exercises

Several basic resistance moves can develop your core strength. I suggest starting with the following exercises: chest press, latissimus pull-down, biceps curl, triceps curl, and reverse fly or row. Some of these exercises not only build shoulder and arm strength but also work the trunk. Doing push-ups is an excellent resistance activity that uses body weight. Figures 4.3 through 4.8 show how to do the exercises with free weights and with tubing or body weight. Machines vary in design, but the names of the exercises usually do not vary.

A common problem with arthritis is loss of handgrip strength. A program that focuses on muscular endurance using low resistance and high repetitions helps tremendously with hand strength. You can buy elaborate devices that are relatively inexpensive through rehabilitation supply companies. You can also use simpler resistance devices, such as hand putty or a soft ball, to work the hand muscles.

Chest Press

The chest press works the pectoral muscles at the front of the upper chest, as well as the triceps. Lie on the ground with your knees bent and your feet flat on the ground. Start with weights in both hands, upper arms on the ground at approximately shoulder level, and elbows bent slightly. Slowly lift the weights toward the sky, bringing your arms together. Lower the weights to the starting position and repeat. If you use tubing, it should be long enough to go under your shoulders as you lie on top of it. The motion is the same as with the free weights. See figure 4.3.

Latissimus Pull-Down

This exercise works your latissimus dorsi, biceps, and pectoralis major. You can perform this movement in sitting or standing position (sitting may make it easier to stabilize), with the tubing behind you, attached to something such as a door, as in figure 4.4. Start with your hands overhead, midway between straight up and straight out. Pull the tubing down and forward until your hands are even with your shoulders. Slowly return to the starting position and repeat.

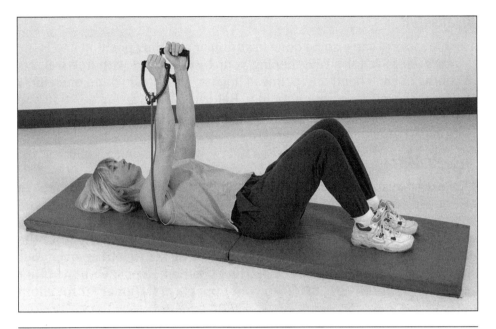

Figure 4.3 Chest press.

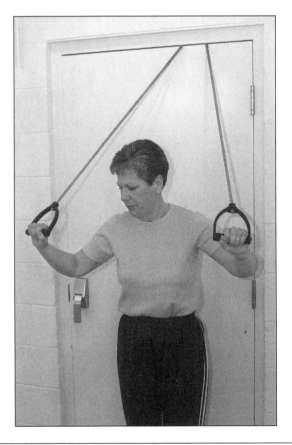

Figure 4.4 Latissimus pull-down.

Biceps Curl

The biceps curl can also be done in sitting or standing position and is the primary exercise for strengthening your biceps. Start with free weights or tubing in each hand and palms facing up, and slowly bend one elbow to bring the weight to your shoulder. Return to the starting position and repeat the motion with the opposite arm. Your upper arm should remain stationary throughout this exercise. See figure 4.5.

Triceps Curl

This exercise strengthens the triceps and is another movement that can be done in sitting or standing position. With your tubing held in one hand behind your back (see figure 4.6), start with the other arm overhead, elbow bent, and hand behind your head, holding the other end of the tubing (or weight). Straighten the elbow to bring the weight up over your shoulder, and then return to the starting position. Repeat with the other arm. As with the biceps curl, keep your upper arm stationary throughout the exercise.

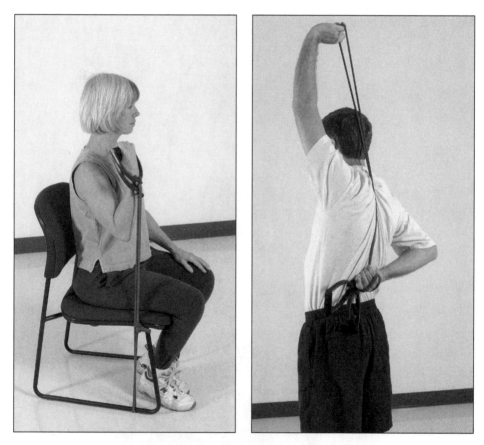

Figure 4.5 Biceps curl.   **Figure 4.6** Triceps curl.

Reverse Fly

A variation of the bent-over lateral raise, this exercise concentrates on the posterior deltoid, rhomboid, and middle trapezius muscles. Stand with your knees bent slightly and bend forward from the hips, keeping your back straight. Hold your free weights in each hand, hanging toward the ground. Raise both weights out to your sides, allowing the elbows to bend slightly (see figure 4.7). Return to the starting position. Be sure to control the movement in both directions.

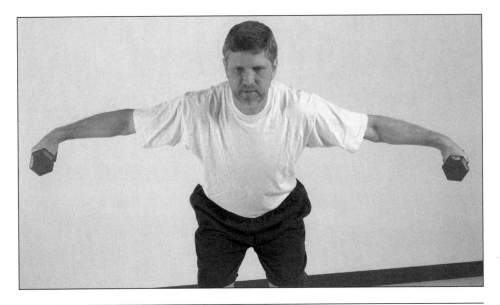

Figure 4.7   Reverse fly.

Row

The row works the same muscles as the reverse fly, and you perform it in a sitting position with tubing. Sitting on the ground with your legs straight out, hook the tubing around your feet. Start with your arms pointing toward your feet, holding the ends of the tubing in both hands. Pull with both arms, bringing your hands towards your shoulders (see figure 4.8). Return to the starting position and repeat.

Abdominal Exercises

Three exercises work the abdominal muscles, each emphasizing different muscle groups. For the abdominal curl-up or crunch, lie on the ground with your knees bent and your feet flat on the ground. Slowly raise your upper trunk off the ground until your shoulder blades clear the floor, with your arms reaching toward your knees (see figure 4.9). Then return to the start position.

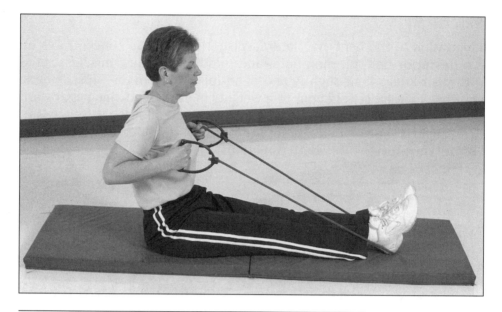

Figure 4.8 Row.

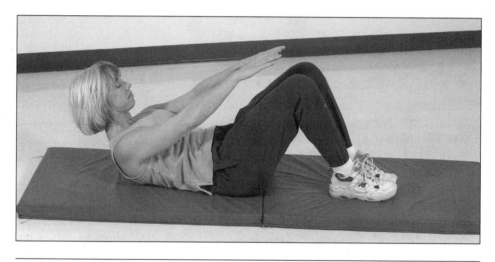

Figure 4.9 Abdominal curl-up.

The pelvic tilt (reverse crunch) also requires you to start on the ground, with your hips and knees bent at a 90-degree angle. Tighten your lower abdominal muscles, attempting to raise your pelvis straight up a few inches (see figure 4.10). Lower your pelvis, then repeat; be sure to keep the hip angle constant.

The last abdominal exercise emphasizes the oblique muscles. Using the same position as for the abdominal crunch, raise your trunk, bringing your left shoulder toward the midline, enough to clear the left shoulder

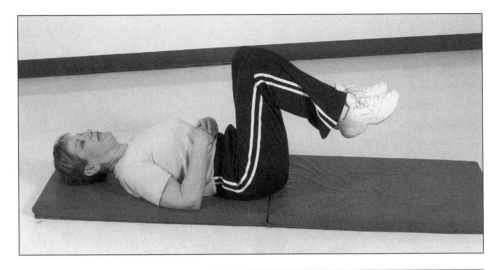

Figure 4.10 Pelvic tilt (reverse crunch).

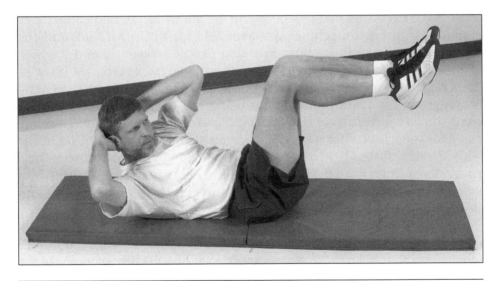

Figure 4.11 Advanced curl-up.

blade (see figure 4.11). Return to the starting position, and then repeat using your right shoulder. Beginners can put their hands at their sides and progress to crossing them over the chest; the most advanced position places the hands behind the neck (do not pull at your neck).

Hand-Strengthening Exercises

The simplest exercise for building grip strength is squeezing a rubber ball or foam device. Once you have developed some hand strength with a ball or soft object, you may be able to work up to a more challenging device such as the one shown in figure 4.12. Make sure that all fingers and the thumb contribute equally to the squeeze to balance the force exerted, and completely relax between squeezes. Also, devices exist that allow you to squeeze one finger at a time so that you can build their strength individually. A simple way to strengthen the finger extensors is to bring all your fingers together and put a rubber band around the ends of the fingers. Then try to spread your fingers.

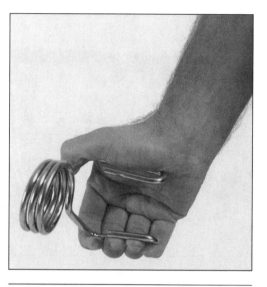

Figure 4.12   Hand-strengthening exercise.

Trunk Exercises

Most of the exercises that I recommend for the trunk are body resistance activities. Although machines are available for both the back and the abdomen, I am cautious about advising people to use them. I have an acquaintance with chronic low back pain who did back stabilization exercises regularly to control the back problem. When she started a strength-training program, she thought that using the back extension machine would further increase her back strength and decrease her pain. The large extensor muscles of her back did become strong, but the motion of the activity exacerbated her back pain. If you decide to try a back machine, I suggest you build a solid base with the body resistance exercises before you advance to the machines; then start with little to no resistance and be especially conscious of proper body position.

As with all resistance activities, you must work opposing muscles, so incorporate both abdominal and back exercises into your program. Emphasize movements that build muscular endurance (although you can increase the resistance for these moves by using handheld weights). A basic program of pelvic tilts and abdominal crunches (see page 91) will do a good job of strengthening the abdomen. Of several exercises for the back, research has suggested that the birddog and the plinth are the most effective (as I note in the section on low back pain at the end of this chapter). A few other back stabilization activities are illustrated to give you some variety in your program and to provide alternatives if you find the first two positions too difficult; they can be uncomfortable on the knees.

Birddog

This exercise primarily builds the muscles that stabilize the spine, although the gluteus maximus, hamstrings, and shoulder girdle muscles also benefit. Start on your hands and knees. Slowly push your right leg back until it is almost straight out; at the same time raise your left arm straight out until it is pointing ahead of you (see figure 4.13). Hold the end position between 10 to 20 seconds and then slowly lower your arm and leg to the start position. Focus on keeping your trunk still during the movement of your arms and legs. Repeat the move with the left leg and right arm.

Plinth

This exercise focuses on the quadratus lumborum, a strong stabilizer of the spine. Start by lying on your side and bending your knees behind you to 90 degrees. Raising your trunk part way off the ground, place your forearm on the ground, with your elbow directly under your shoulder. Next, lift your hips off the ground until your body is in a straight line. An easy way to picture this position is to think of your upper arm and body as two sides of a triangle, with the ground being the third side (see figure 4.14). Hold this position 10 to 20 seconds and then slowly lower your hips back to the ground. Repeat on the opposite side. To perform the advanced plinth, use your feet as the axis on the ground, rather than your knee.

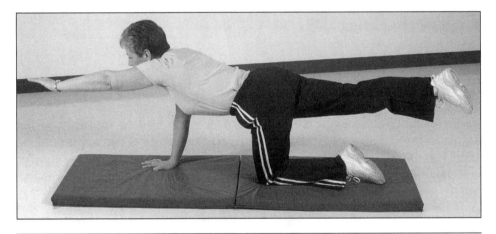

Figure 4.13 Birddog.

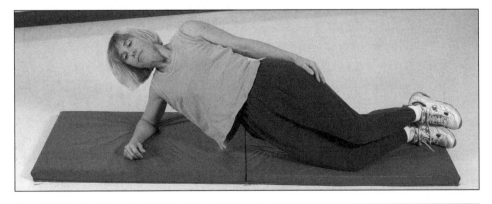

Figure 4.14 Plinth.

Bridge for Back Stabilization

This position uses the erector spinae and the hip extensors. Start in a lying position with your knees bent and your feet flat on the ground. Lift your hips straight off the ground until your trunk and thighs are in a straight line and hold for 10 to 20 seconds (see figure 4.15). Slowly return to the starting position.

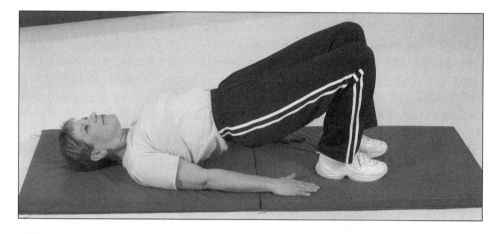

Figure 4.15 Bridge for back stabilization.

Cat-Camel

The cat-camel is an exercise that helps provide limited mobility to the spine and thus improves nutrition to the intervertebral discs. Starting on your hands and knees, gently sag and then arch your back (see figures 4.16, a and b). Both movements should be controlled and not excessive in either direction. Repeat the action several times.

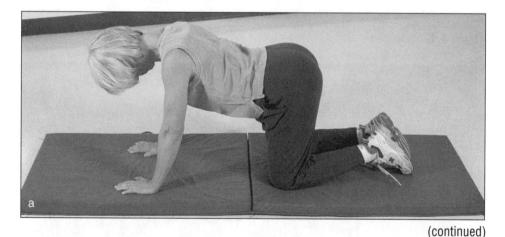

(continued)

Figure 4.16 Cat-camel.

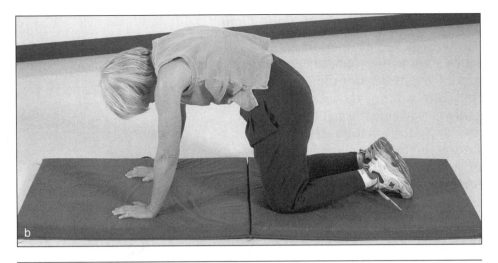

Figure 4.16 *(continued).*

Lower Body Exercises

Lower body strength is very important for function and for reduction of knee and hip pain. If you emphasize any one area of strengthening, this may be the most crucial one. The leg press is probably the most common of the exercises; a routine that includes hip extension, abduction and adduction, and hamstring curls will greatly improve mobility and stability. At home you can perform wall squats using your body weight. All of these exercises can be performed with cuff weights or tubing. I have patients whose tubing I had to replace because they used it so much that it finally snapped.

Leg Press, Closed Chain

This exercise strengthens the quadriceps and gluteal muscles. Stand with your feet about shoulder width apart, with tubing placed under your feet. Bend your hips and knees slightly and grasp the tubing so there is slight tension (see figure 4.17). Keeping your back straight, straighten your hips and knees and come to a complete standing position. Slowly lower yourself to the starting position and repeat.

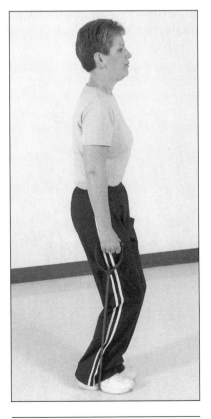

Figure 4.17 Leg press, closed chain.

Leg Flexion and Extension, Open Chain

These exercises are performed in a sitting position, and they work the hamstrings and the quadriceps, respectively. Secure one end of your tubing around a table leg or other stable item that will not move and the other end around the ankle on the side that you want to exercise. For flexion the tubing will be in front of you, and it will be behind you for extension. To perform an extension, start with one knee bent (the leg without the tubing) so that your foot is slightly under you. Extend the knee of the leg with the tubing so that your foot moves away from you (see figure 4.18a), and hold at the end of the motion 2 to 3 seconds. Then bring your foot back in a controlled motion. For flexion, slowly bring your foot toward you and hold in the same manner as before (see figure 4.18b).

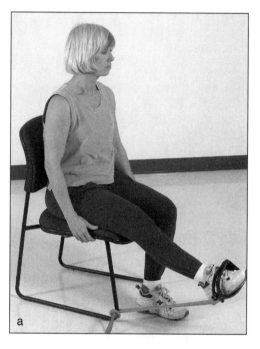

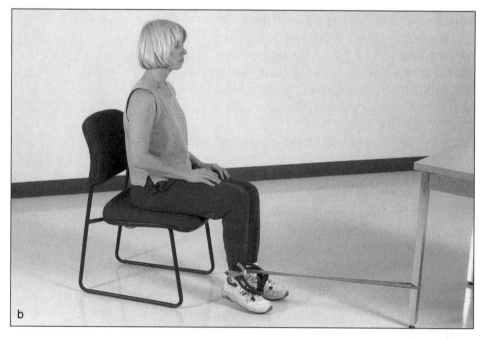

Figure 4.18 (a) Leg extension and (b) leg flexion, open chain.

Hip Extension and Flexion, Open Chain

Hip extension focuses on the gluteal and hamstring muscles, while the hip flexion exercise stresses the iliopsoas and quadriceps muscles. Because one stands to do both exercises, other hip stabilizers also work. As with the knee exercises, secure one end of your tubing to a stable object and the other end just below the knee. For extension, face the tubing and keep your body erect and knee fairly straight. Move your thigh backward so that the movement is taking place at your hip (see figure 4.19a). For flexion, turn so you are facing away from the tubing and bring your thigh forward (figure 4.19b). Hold at the end position for 2 to 3 seconds, then repeat.

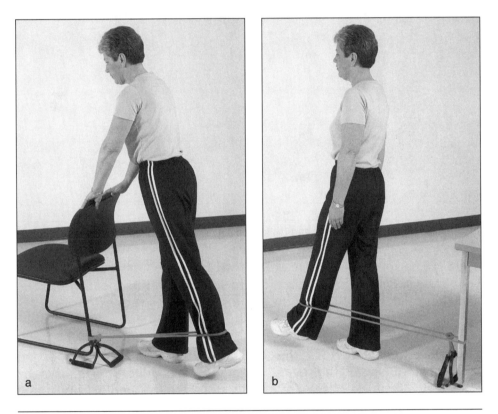

Figure 4.19   (a) Hip extension and (b) hip flexion, open chain.

Knee Extension and Flexion, Closed Chain

These exercises are another way of working the quadriceps and hamstrings. As with the hip exercises, you do these while standing, with the tubing attached to a stable object and just above your knee. For extension, face the tubing and slightly bend the knee on which the tubing is tied (figure 4.20a). Straighten your knee into the resistance and hold this straightened position for 2 to 3 seconds before letting your knee bend

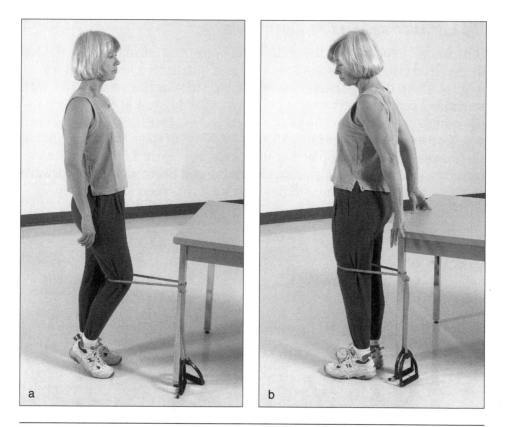

Figure 4.20 (a) Knee extension and (b) knee flexion, closed chain.

again. To perform knee flexion, turn away from the tubing and start with your knee in a straight position (figure 4.20b). You then bend your knee into the resistance, following the same sequence as with extension.

Hip Abduction and Adduction

The primary hip abductor is the gluteus medius, which is very important for normal walking. Of the several adductors, the adductor magnus is the strongest. These exercises are usually done while standing, but if you have a loop of tubing, you can do the abduction from a side-lying position. As with the other standing exercises, secure one end of your tubing to an immobile object and the other end to the ankle of the leg you will be moving. For hip abduction, stand sideways to the stable object so that your feet are together and the moving leg is farther away from the object. Move the leg sideways, away from your body and against the resistance (see figure 4.21a). To perform hip adduction, the moving leg is on the side of the body closest to the stable object. This time bring the leg across your body, in front of the other leg, as it pulls against the tubing (figure 4.21b). In both exercises, hold the end-point position for 2 to 3 seconds, and then return the leg to its starting position.

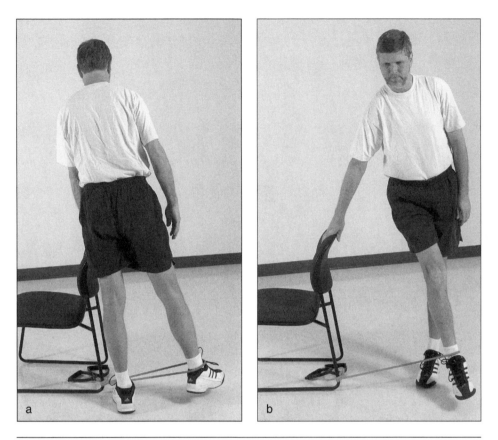

Figure 4.21 (a) Hip abduction and (b) adduction.

Hip Internal and External Rotation

These exercises work the respective rotators of the hip and are easiest to do while sitting. To perform internal rotation, secure one end of the tubing around the ankle of the moving leg and the other end to the leg of the chair on the side of your other leg (see figure 4.22a). Bring your foot away from your body while you roll your thigh inward. For external rotation, attach the tubing to one ankle and the leg of the chair nearest that ankle. Bring your foot across, in front of the other foot, while the knee rolls outward (see figure 4.22b). Again, hold the end position for 2 to 3 seconds before returning to your starting position. With both exercises, allow only rotation of the thigh, and not adduction or abduction.

Sample Programs

I have outlined two types of sample programs—one for use with machines at a health club, and the other for use with equipment at home. I have drawn up two examples of the machine resistance program. The first is

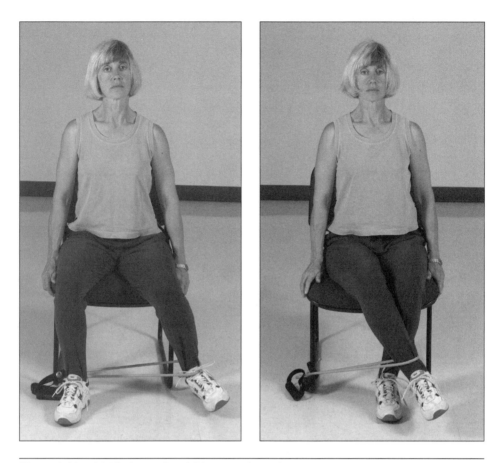

Figure 4.22 (a) Hip internal and (b) external rotation.

suitable for a beginner (see table 4.2) and the second for someone who already possesses some strength (see table 4.3). The primary difference between the two levels is intensity; the individual who is already doing a program can begin at a higher resistance.

The beginner starts at a low intensity for two primary reasons. First, a beginner is less likely to develop extreme soreness with a low-intensity program and therefore is more likely to want to come back for another round. Second, low intensity gives one's tissues a chance to adapt to the overloads more gradually, so the exercises are less likely to aggravate arthritis.

For the advanced person, I have drawn up a program with three sets and a resistance level of 80 percent of 1RM; you would modify this regimen to fit your own goals. One set yields satisfactory improvements in strength and takes less time. If you want to develop greater muscular endurance, keep the resistance at about 70 percent of your 1RM and increase the number of repetitions to 10 or more.

Table 4.2   Initial Resistance Program With Machines for Beginner

Frequency	Intensity	Repetitions	Sets	Exercises
2 times/week	50% of 1RM	10	1	Chest presses, biceps curls, lat pull-downs, rows, hip extensions, leg presses, hamstring curls, hip abductions

Table 4.3   Advanced Resistance Program With Machines and Free Weights

Frequency	Intensity	Repetitions	Sets	Exercises
3 times/week	80% of 1RM	8-10	1-3	Chest presses, biceps curls, lat pull-downs, rows, overhead presses, hip extensions, leg presses, hamstring curls, hip abduction, reverse flys

Home programs for the beginner and the already active person are also very similar, so I have only shown a beginner program (table 4.4). The primary difference is once again the intensity; the beginner starts with lighter tubing or free weights. In addition, a beginner does 10 to 15 repetitions of an activity for one set, eventually working up to three sets, while a more advanced person can start at three sets. Both need to progress the amount of resistance in due course if they wish to keep improving their strength.

As part of either a home- or facility-based program, you should include trunk exercises. A well-balanced program includes abdominal curls and back stabilization exercises. Most people can start with two to three sets of 10 repetitions for the curls, gradually increasing to 20 repetitions. The back stabilization exercises are isometric holds; move to the end position

Table 4.4   Home Exercise Program for Beginner

Frequency	Intensity	Repetitions	Sets	Exercises
3 times/week	Moderate	10-15	1	Rows, biceps curls, triceps curls, chest presses, push-ups, hip extensions, wall squats, hamstring flexions, abdominal curls

and maintain it for 10 to 30 seconds (recommendations differ on the hold times, so I have suggested a range). The main concern is that the holds do not cause pain. Repeat each hold 5 to 10 times. As I mention in the upcoming section on pain, you may find it most comfortable to alternate between back and abdominal exercises.

Energy for Training

The goal of preactivity food intake is to provide energy for the upcoming session while minimizing stomach distress. Here are some guidelines:

▷ Eat a small amount of easily digested carbohydrates (such as a muffin, bagel, or granola bar) about 1 hour before an intense exercise session.

▷ Drink a carbohydrate or electrolyte replacement fluid during longer, high-intensity sessions, or water during short sessions.

▷ After an exercise session, rehydrate as soon as possible.

▷ After an intense session, eat an easily digested carbohydrate (fruit or one of the foods listed earlier).

Precautions

Resistance training, like any physical activity, entails some risks; but proper techniques and safety precautions can reduce those risks. Before beginning your resistance-training program, familiarize yourself with a few safety concepts.

Valsalva Maneuver

One problem that can occur with resistance training relates to holding one's breath. Many people hold their breath when they are lifting a heavy weight, thereby increasing the amount of force they can produce. They are trying to exhale against a closed windpipe, an attempt that creates increased pressure in the trunk. This pressure stabilizes the trunk, allowing one to produce more force for a given movement. The technique is called the Valsalva maneuver. This maneuver causes an extremely rapid rise in blood pressure, which is followed by a fall in arterial blood pressure. The result is dizziness, blurred vision, and sometimes fainting. To avoid potential problems, concentrate on exhaling slowly while doing your resistance movement. You might practice a pattern of breathing in just before the lift, breathing out slowly through pursed lips during the lift, and breathing in again while you return to your starting position.

Hypertension

If you have high blood pressure but your blood pressure is under control, you can participate safely in resistance training as part of a complete exercise program. Check with your physician before starting any program; once you are cleared, you can begin. I recommend checking your blood pressure each time you prepare to do your resistance-training program. If your resting blood pressure starts to rise, let your physician know immediately and reduce your strength training temporarily. Recommendations for individuals with hypertension emphasize using high repetition and low resistance in the program. Circuit training is a viable option for those with hypertension.

Low Back Pain

Low back pain is one of the most common complaints that physicians and therapists treat, and epidemiological studies suggest that as many as 85 percent of adults will have back pain at some time. Strength training is part of a program to reduce back pain, but some moves may exacerbate low back pain. Moves that require repeated trunk twisting or extension and flexion may cause problems with your low back. If you have already had back problems, you may want to avoid such moves. Some of the back extension equipment in gyms, although good for strengthening, may promote too much movement in the spine and thus increase your pain.

Exercises that strengthen the back in a neutral position may be best for controlling chronic back pain. These exercises are usually called back stabilization exercises; they involve movements that keep the trunk and spine stationary while moving the arms, legs, or both.

Two exercises are especially effective for stabilizing the spine without putting undue pressure on it during the activity (McGill 2001). These exercises are the birddog and the plinth, previously described in the section on trunk exercises (see page 92). Most therapists suggest holding each position for 10 to 20 seconds (you may need to work up to this duration) and repeating the activity 5 times. Before doing these stabilization exercises, perform the cat-camel exercise (on page 94) 6 to 8 times to gently mobilize your spine.

I find that I am most comfortable when I alternate some of the back exercises with some of the abdominal exercises. The abdominal exercises help to stretch the back without overstretching it. I do both the back and abdominal exercises either after my cardiovascular workout or at the end of the day. Back stabilization exercises are designed to build muscular endurance in the small muscles surrounding the spine, so do them daily.

Personalizing Your Program

Just as you do with aerobic exercise and with your program as a whole, design your strength-training routine to meet your needs. When I set up my strength program, I had two broad goals: strengthening my hips and knees so that I could run, and building my upper body strength and endurance to help improve my golf game. I visit the university gym two days a week to work out, although I have an alternate home program for the days when I cannot get there. Because running is an endurance activity and because I have chronic knee problems, I use slightly lower resistance (about 60 percent) and more repetitions (two sets of 15 reps). I also do back stabilization and abdominal exercises daily. The only difficulty I have is controlling my competitive urges; if a young woman is before me on a machine, I find myself checking out how much weight she is lifting and comparing it to my own lifts. Luckily, I can control urges to try more, even if my ego wants to. If you are competitive, remind yourself that training should not be a competition.

A woman with whom I worked had a primary goal of decreasing her knee pain so that she could walk regularly. She does a home program using cuff weights three times weekly. Her routine includes single leg lifts, side leg lifts (abduction), and biceps curls. She does one set of 10 partial squats, followed by abdominal and back exercises. Once she reached a level at which she was not having knee pain, she maintained her program at that level rather than progressing it further. A young man I know of also likes to keep his strength program at home. He concentrates on abdominal work (200 sit-ups per day) and upper body work (100 push-ups each day, despite his shoulder arthritis).

Other people have told me they prefer a gym. One gentleman started out with some free weights and upper-body exercises at home. When he felt that his strength was adequate, he switched to a local facility. His program is simple—he does one set of 10 repetitions for each lift, performing most of the lifts that I suggested earlier. This type of program is short and easier to fit into a busy schedule.

Although some of you may feel that strength training is for athletes, I maintain that it is for all of us. Throughout this chapter I point out some of the ways that building muscular strength can help decrease the stress and pain of arthritis and enhance your ability to participate in the activities you enjoy. Use the information presented in this chapter to design your own resistance-training program.

The final component of an exercise program is flexibility, which I will discuss in detail in chapter 5. As I stated earlier, this topic is especially relevant to arthritis; one of the hallmarks of arthritis is the loss of one's flexibility and range of motion. You can decrease both of these problems by incorporating some very simple activities into your daily schedule.

ACTION PLAN:
BUILDING A STRENGTH PROGRAM

- ☐ Decide whether you want to focus on muscular endurance, pure strength, or both.
- ☐ Determine your intensity (based on a percentage of your 1-, 6-, or 10-lift maximum or on your body weight).
- ☐ Design your progression.
- ☐ Set your frequency (recommendation is 2 to 3 days per week).
- ☐ Understand the types of muscle contraction (concentric, eccentric, and isometric) and the difference between open chain and closed chain exercises.
- ☐ Consider logistics such as whether to exercise at home or at a gym.
- ☐ Use the sample programs and the exercises in this chapter to develop a program based on your needs and goals.

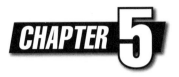

CHAPTER 5

PURSUING PAIN-FREE FLEXIBILITY

B ecause stiffness is one of the hallmarks of arthritis, flexibility is a crucial component of your exercise program. Arthritis patients tend to limit movement because of pain and stiffness; they lose both flexibility and joint motion as one of the earliest results of such restriction. Once again, the notion that if you don't move it (a muscle or joint), it won't hurt does not apply to arthritis. If you do not move an involved joint, muscular tightness increases and joint motion is lost. The joint becomes stiffer and more painful—the exact opposite of what you want. The lost range of movement can only be restored by stretching the tight muscles. Regular motion of each joint leads to a decrease in stiffness and an associated reduction in pain. I cannot guarantee pain-free motion, but you can significantly diminish pain and stiffness with a regular flexibility program.

The benefits of flexibility are even more evident in the context of a total exercise program. Studies have connected proper flexibility to reduced potential for muscle injury, decreased low back pain, and better biomechanics. Other benefits of a regular stretching program include reduced anxiety and lower blood pressure. Stretching and range of motion activities are components of well-designed warm-up and cool-down periods.

An elderly lady I know had arthritis in her hands, hips, and knees. Although she did not have a formal stretching program, whenever she started to feel stiff, she would do some gentle range of motion exercises. She said this practice especially helped her hands and enabled her to keep up hobbies like crocheting. Even at 90 years of age, she had no loss of motion in her hips or knees, which meant she could dress, bathe, and do other activities that are often compromised when joint motion is decreased. The exercise habits she had developed much earlier in her life allowed her to keep active and enjoy her later years.

One young man, only 31 years old, reported that he had started having serious problems with his shoulders while still in high school. He was a competitive swimmer and did lots of heavy weightlifting; he was diagnosed at that time with osteoarthritis. After finishing high school, he decreased the weightlifting and started doing range of motion exercises for his shoulders, under the direction of a physical therapist. He has now combined his flexibility work with regular aerobic exercise and a resistance program that uses body weight. He still does the same range of motion routine and is virtually free of pain. Even when he does have pain, he is able to control it with Tylenol and glucosamine. He is able to maintain full range of motion in his shoulders, except during very wet weather.

Flexibility and joint range can be restored if the loss is temporary, but the longer the impairment lasts, the more difficult it will be to regain your motion. Therefore you need to get started on this an aspect of your program, even if you do not currently have any loss in motion. Remember the adage, "An ounce of prevention is worth a pound of cure." Every year patients are referred to physical therapy for treatment of "frozen shoulder," a loss of motion in the shoulder that occurs when parts of the joint capsule adhere to one another. Many of these patients could have avoided a trip to therapy if they had maintained their upper extremity activity. The most common factor leading to this problem is shoulder pain, which causes the person to stop moving the shoulder. Instead of ceasing all motion, modify the activities you are doing, see your physician, and implement a strengthening and flexibility program.

Generalized Versus Specific Flexibility

One can think of flexibility either as the general ability to move in a combination of ways, or as the particular ability to move one or two joints in a specific motion. For example, chapter 1 mentioned a generalized test of shoulder flexibility, the Apley's scratch test. The object of the test is to bring the hands together in the middle of the back, one hand reaching from below and the other from above. This movement uses internal rotation, extension, and adduction together for one shoulder, while the other uses a different combination of motions.

You use combined motion in many functional activities that require general flexibility, such as combing your hair or tucking your shirt in at the back. Sometimes a person cannot perform a combined movement because of loss of motion in one specific direction. If you cannot move your arm above the level of your shoulder, you lack one component of the combined movement and thus do not have general flexibility. Often one loses a little bit from each type of movement that contributes to the total motion.

As you determine your needs, decide if you need general or specific flexibility; most people need some of each. Chapter 2 mentioned two generalized tests of flexibility. Specific flexibility is usually measured by a health care provider using a special tool called a goniometer, which quantifies the range of motion for a joint.

If you have severe limitations, I suggest you see a therapist who can assess your specific needs and help you determine realistic goals. It may be necessary to set a goal that aims for less than complete range of motion but facilitates function. For example, in a previous chapter I discussed a patient who had lost significant motion in her shoulder and could not touch the top of her head. Because of her age and the degeneration in her shoulder joint, we set a goal that would make it possible for her to lift her hand to the top of her head. We did not try for the ability to reach her arm straight up from her shoulder; she did not need that much motion and was unlikely to attain it.

Conditions Affecting Flexibility and Response to Stretching

Although much of the body's response to stretching is neural, several factors affect both one's flexibility and one's response to range of motion and stretching activities. You can modify some of these elements but not all. Factors you cannot change are age, presence of disease, previous injury to the muscle or joint, and scar tissue. You can, however, alter temperature and muscle imbalance, which influence a person's flexibility and response to stretching.

As tissue temperature rises, elasticity increases, and vice versa—as temperature drops, flexibility decreases. This change in flexibility can be as much as 20 percent of the original range of motion. This relationship explains why you feel stiffer when you are cold and why keeping your muscles warm while exercising in the cold is essential. It also suggests methods for improving one's flexibility and response to stretching activities. We can warm tissues by internal means, muscle contractions, or external means. External ways of increasing tissue temperature are as simple as covering the joint, applying heat packs, or taking a warm shower. One friend uses a neoprene sleeve for his knee when it is cold outside. He reports that not only does the sleeve keep the swelling down in his knee, but the warmth helps him feel looser and decreases the pain.

The strength of the muscles on either side of the joint, or in some cases adjacent to the joint, affects its range of motion. Around each joint opposing muscles create a sort of balance. If these muscles are sufficiently strong and flexible, they allow the joint to move through its entire range. However, if one set of muscles becomes weak compared to the opposing set, joint motion may be compromised. Poor posture and tight muscles can worsen such an imbalance.

For example, a common imbalance is one between the anterior and posterior shoulder muscles. Most of the time people perform tasks and lift objects in front of their bodies; as a result, the anterior muscles become stronger than the posterior ones. Habitually poor posture (such as hunching forward with rounded shoulders) exacerbates this condition. Poor posture combined with the muscle imbalance leads to tight pectoral muscles (although it is not really possible to say which of these problems comes first). Limited range of motion and shoulder pain are usually the consequences of these deficits. Although this chapter covers only flexibility, you can see how all of the components of fitness are interrelated.

Special Issues Related to Stretching

▷ Because of muscular stiffness, you may need to further warm muscles before stretching. A warm shower or heat packs help improve your muscles' response to stretching.

▷ Although losing range of motion is the most common problem with arthritis, you may actually have too much motion at some joints because of changes in ligaments. Make sure you do not stretch beyond the normal range of movement.

▷ As one ages, muscles lose some of their water, which decreases their elasticity. Make sure you stay hydrated to keep your muscles pliable.

▷ For extremely stiff and inflexible muscles, you may find that a prolonged stretch (1 to 5 minutes) produces more results. Be sure to find a relaxed, comfortable position.

▷ Range of motion activities done in warm water, such as one performs in aquatics classes, are both fun and effective.

Stretching and Flexibility Techniques

The common stretching techniques include static, ballistic, PNF (proprioceptive neuromuscular facilitation), and active isolated stretching. Active range of motion, though not a form of stretching, is a flexibility technique that helps to maintain normal movement in a joint. You may hear about other sorts of stretching; most of them are variations of these techniques. Even though I do not necessarily recommend all of these methods, you should know a little about each type of stretch. A brief description of each can help you decide which technique is most applicable to your situation.

Static Stretching

Static stretching is probably the easiest and most useful to do. I like to prescribe static stretching as part of a program; it is not only simple but relaxing, and you do not need assistance to do it. A static stretch entails moving into a position where you feel a gentle pull on the muscle that you wish to stretch and then holding that position. As the muscle relaxes, you can usually stretch it slightly more, and with each subsequent stretch your range will improve.

A 30-second stretch is the most effective, and 3 to 5 repetitions of that stretch yield the greatest improvements (Bandy, Irion, and Briggler 1997; Bandy, Irion, and Briggler 1998). The time frame for smaller muscles may be slightly less, but I recommend sticking with a 30-second stretch for any muscles that are stiff. Stretch at least three times per week; I recommend stretching daily. Improvements are rapidly lost after cessation of a stretching program, and a daily program will help reduce your stiffness.

Ballistic Stretching

Ballistic stretching employs a repetitive bouncing motion to induce a stretch. Although often defined as a high-intensity activity, variations in speed affect the intensity (several studies use the term "gentle bounce" to describe the appropriate movement). Ballistic stretching has received a bad reputation, based mostly on theory and not on any research. Numerous authors suggest that the chance of pulling a muscle increases when performing a ballistic stretch. Perhaps the risk is greater if one performs a vigorous ballistic motion without having warmed up the muscle, but a few studies have shown ballistic stretching produces gains in flexibility that are similar to those achieved by static stretching, without any negative side effects (Millar and Nephew 1999; Arakawa, Olewe, and Millar 2002; unpublished studies).

The key to using ballistic stretching properly is to warm up with mild aerobic activity and then use a gentle (not vigorous) bouncing motion. The time and repetition guidelines are the same as for static stretching—30 seconds, 3 to 5 repetitions. I only recommend it as a warm-up activity for those of you who do not have a great deal of stiffness, however, because little information is available on how arthritis patients respond to ballistic stretching. The stiffer your muscles are, the greater the probability that they will not respond favorably to a ballistic stretch.

Proprioceptive Neuromuscular Facilitation (PNF)

Proprioceptive neuromuscular facilitation (PNF) is a technique that uses nervous system reflexes to help relax a muscle. For example, as you contract your quadriceps, the opposite muscle (hamstring) relaxes to allow normal motion of the knee joint. One PNF method requires you to contract your quadriceps against a resistance and then relax, while a stretch is applied to the hamstring (see figure 5.1). Although highly effective, these stretches require a partner and rely heavily on appropriate technique (Sady, Wortman, and Blanke 1982). I usually recommend these types of stretches for more athletically inclined individuals who are working with a team. Even if such is the case, make sure to perform the techniques properly. The resistance is not meant to be overpowering, and the stretch should be tolerable.

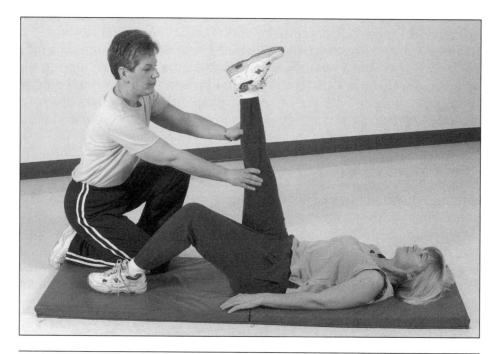

Figure 5.1 PNF stretch for the hamstrings.

Active Isolated Stretching

Active isolated stretching is a relatively new variation of assisted stretching that has grown in popularity in the last few years. Although there is little research on the topic, the studies that do exist find it to be an effective method. This technique combines a short static stretch (with an active contraction of the opposing muscle) with assistance in the direction of the stretch, usually in the form of a rope. The duration for this type of stretch is usually 2 seconds, with 6 to 8 repetitions, although I have seen several variations on the length of hold (Wharton and Wharton 1996).

This stretching technique appears to be simpler to perform than PNF stretching, and many individuals like it because of the shorter duration. Whether or not active isolated stretching is effective for persons with arthritis has not been examined, and I urge caution if you decide to try it; the use of an assistive device can lead some people to be overly aggressive with their stretching. Overstretching can cause muscle damage and may decrease the stability around your joints. On the positive side, if your schedule is limited, your stretching session is much shorter with this type of program.

Active Range of Motion

Active range of motion is a flexibility technique commonly used by physical therapists as part of rehabilitation programs. It is not actually a method of stretching but is used to promote normal motion. Active range of motion exercises have been employed successfully with individuals who have rheumatoid arthritis (Byers 1985), and they are easy to perform. These activities involve using the muscles that surround a joint to move the joint completely through its available range of motion. An example is opening and closing your hand, making sure that you completely extend and flex all of the fingers each time. For the best results, a range of motion exercise should be performed 5 to 10 times, depending on comfort (Kisner and Colby 2002). You do not have to hold the position at either end of the motion, nor do you use any resistance.

You can perform these exercises as assisted activities by using pulleys, a cane, or any other device that helps you move the joint throughout its range. Since range of motion activities are not truly stretches, they are most useful for maintaining normal range and decreasing stiffness in a joint, whereas the previous activities are designed to actually increase the joint's range of motion. A benefit especially important to arthritis patients is that these movements load and unload the joint, a process that helps nutritional substances get into a joint and metabolic byproducts get out of it (Goodman and Boissonnault 2003).

Adding Flexibility to Your Daily Routine

When deciding which type of flexibility activities to use, you must consider the severity of your arthritis and your personal needs. I recommend using both the static stretching technique and active range of motion activities (see table 5.1 for guidelines). These two methods tend to be easier to do properly, and you do not need a partner or any special equipment. You need both—static stretches focus on increasing flexibility and loosen up muscles that are tight or motions that are restricted, whereas range of motion activities maintain normal motion.

Do active range of motion exercises daily. Range of motion activities are a good way to get started in the morning; you can even intersperse them throughout the day for joints that tend to stiffen quickly. Since moist heat helps increase circulation to your muscles and decrease stiffness, a warm shower is a good place to do some easy motion activities (if you have

Table 5.1   Stretching Guidelines

Static stretch	Active range of motion
Duration: hold 30 seconds	Frequency: 5-10 repetitions
Repetitions: 3-5 per stretch	Intensity: gentle
Intensity: gentle	Motion: continuous, controlled

room). Or you can do your routine just after coming out of the shower. Do a few repetitions after being still for long periods, such as after a daily rest or when you have been sitting for a prolonged time. Gentle range of motion in the evening, before retiring, may lessen morning stiffness. You may also find a simple flexibility routine a nice way to relax at the end of the day.

Static stretches work well as part of your cool-down routine after your aerobic or strength activities. You can vary the stretches according to the activity you are focusing on, such as working on legs for the days you are walking. On days when you have done strength training, add a few upper-extremity and lower-extremity stretches. I also tell patients that static stretches are good for when they're relaxing in front of the television, if they have problems with tightness. For example, many people have very tight hamstrings, perhaps from sitting so much. At the end of the day, if you are watching some television, break up your sitting time by getting on the floor and doing your stretches.

Range of Motion Activities

Several simple movements are good general flexibility exercises and can be interspersed, as I said earlier, with other activities throughout the day. Follow the guidelines for active range of motion: 5 to 10 repetitions using a continuous, controlled motion, within the available range of movement.

For those of us who work at a desk or do a lot of reading and writing, the shoulders, neck, and hands need some regular movement. You can do several activities while sitting, although getting up and moving around on a regular basis is a good way to reduce or prevent total body stiffness. Shoulder rolls are an excellent way to mobilize the muscles around the shoulder. After loosening up your shoulders, gently stretch your neck. Finally, open and close your hands a few times to relax your fingers. A friend of mine was having problems with wrist and hand pain after working at the computer. I suggested she add these simple activities into her workday, doing them every hour (she set an alarm on her computer to remind her). Within one week she no longer had wrist or hand pain, and she found that the short breaks also helped her concentration.

One simple activity is a version of reaching for the sky that enhances shoulder and trunk flexibility. Another way to perform some trunk rotation and combined shoulder movement is a variation of a technique that physical therapists use—the diagonal shoulder stretch, which a colleague of mine used to call the "Vanna White" move. You can do either of these moves (with some modification) in a chair

Daily Range of Motion Activities

▷ Sky stretch

▷ Shoulder rolls

▷ Wrist and hand movements

▷ Modified cycle motion for legs

during the workday or when you have difficulty standing for a lengthy period. A description of both movements follows.

Sky Stretch

Stand with your feet about shoulder width apart. Place one hand on your hip and reach towards the sky with the other hand. Continue to bring your arm over your head and arch your torso slightly in the same direction as the reach (see figure 5.2). Alternate sides, repeating the sequence.

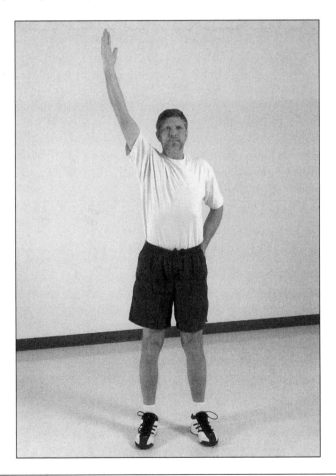

Figure 5.2   Sky stretch.

Diagonal Shoulder Stretch

Stand with your feet about shoulder width apart and your hips facing straight ahead. Put one hand on the opposite hip bone and turn your shoulders slightly in the direction of that hip (see figure 5.3a). From this position, roll the palm of your hand forward, and in a smooth, continuous motion, describe an arc with your arm. End the motion with your arm and shoulder pointing up and back (see figure 5.3b). Repeat this movement on the other side.

Modified Shoulder Stretch in Sitting

While sitting, lean forward and to the left, bringing your right arm toward your left ankle. Roll your hand forward, leading the right arm in a large arc toward the sky, which will end behind your right side, with your trunk twisting slightly to the right. Repeat this movement with your left arm.

Shoulder Rolls

Bring your shoulders forward, up, slowly back, down, and then together, with your shoulder blades toward the spine. Hold your shoulders at the end position for a few seconds before starting a second roll.

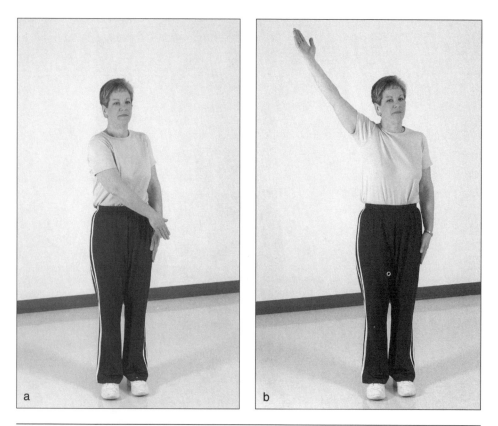

Figure 5.3 Diagonal shoulder stretch.

Neck Stretch

Bring your right ear toward your right shoulder, holding for 5 to 10 seconds at the point where you feel a gentle stretch (see figure 5.4). Then slowly bring your left ear toward the other shoulder, repeating the hold. The emphasis here is on gentle, pain-free motion.

Hand Range of Motion

Close both hands into fists, then open them as wide as possible. Another movement is to close and open your fingers in a fanning motion, starting with the little finger and ending with your thumb.

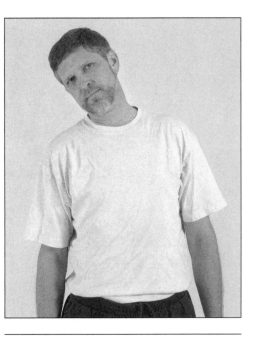

Figure 5.4   Neck stretch.

Cycling Range of Motion

A good flexibility activity for the lower body is a modified cycling motion. This exercise works both the hips and the knees, and you can do it in modified form while standing and holding on to a support.

Lying on your back, take one leg at a time through a cycling motion. Slide your foot along the ground toward your buttock, then raise your knee toward your chest, and finally extend your leg back out to the starting position (see figure 5.5). Repeat this sequence with the opposite leg.

Sitting Hip Rotation

Hip rotation often declines when arthritis is present in the hip. You can perform rotation exercises in a sitting position, which may be easier, but with adequate support you can do them standing.

While sitting in a chair with your knees bent, slide your left foot back so the right leg can move to the left without interference. Swing your lower right leg like a pendulum, from side to side, with the knee and thigh acting as the axis of rotation (see figure 5.6). Repeat this movement with the left leg.

Ankle Range of Motion

Finish off your range of motion activities for the lower body with some ankle movements, such as circles. While sitting down, slowly describe a circle with your foot, first a few times in one direction, then a few times in the opposite direction. End the move by flexing your ankle; bring the top of the foot toward the front of the leg. Repeat this sequence with your other ankle.

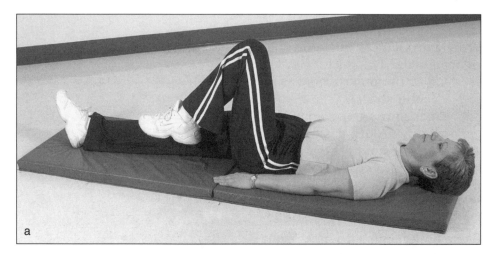

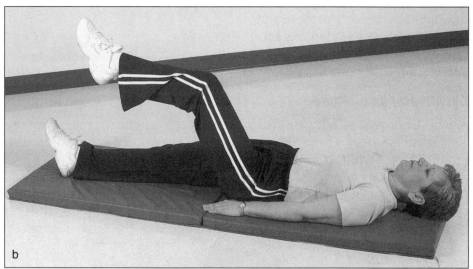

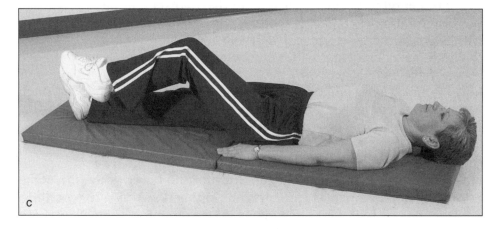

Figure 5.5 Cycling range of motion.

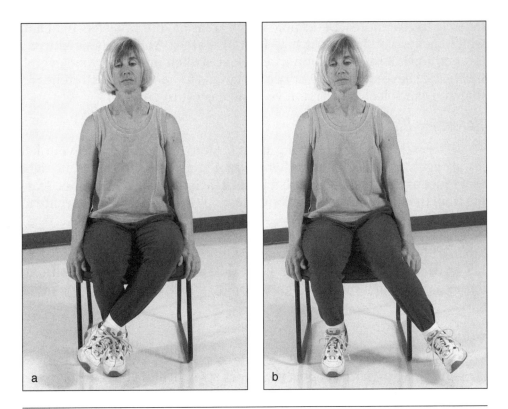

Figure 5.6 Sitting hip rotation.

Specific Stretching Activities

There are stretches for almost every muscle or group of muscles in your body, but I have concentrated on areas that have a tendency to become tight and can limit motion. These areas include the hips, hamstrings, calves, and anterior shoulders. You only need to stretch those areas that are tight; for the rest you can do range of motion activities. As I indicated earlier, use a static stretch for these tight muscles—three to five stretches per muscle group, with a 30-second hold per stretch. You should feel a gentle pull, and the stretch should not increase pain in the joint or muscle. I suggest doing these stretches as part of your cool-down after aerobic exercise.

A good way to organize your stretching routine is to do all of your sitting stretches and then your standing stretches. It may be less boring if you do only the first repetition of each stretch, in a series, and then repeat the series. For example, start with a hamstring stretch, transition to a groin (adductor muscle) stretch, next do a rotator (piriformis) stretch on each side, and then repeat the sequence. After you do three to five of these sitting stretches, move to a standing position and stretch your hip flexors and calf muscles. Doing all of these movements, with 30-second holds, takes 15 to 20 minutes. Determine which areas of your body feel tight and which moves you find most help for those areas. You rarely need to do 5 repetitions; 3 reps give you a sufficient stretch and help your overall flexibility. I have shown one or two variations for most of the stretches so that you can select the version you find easiest to perform.

Hamstring Stretches

To perform the sitting hamstring stretch, sit on the ground with your left leg straight in front of you and your right knee bent, so that your right foot touches the inside of your left knee. Reach toward your left foot, leaning from the hips and keeping your chest up (see figure 5.7). Alternate to stretch the right hamstring.

You can also stretch your hamstring from a lying position. Bend your hip to a 90–degree angle and interlock your fingers behind that thigh, just below the knee. Then straighten your knee as much as possible without letting your thigh move (see figure 5.8). Repeat this stretch on the other side.

Groin Stretch

While sitting, spread your legs as wide as possible, keeping your knees straight. Lean forward, keeping your back straight and your chest up (see figure 5.9). You can include the hamstrings by stretching to each side after you have performed the move to the center.

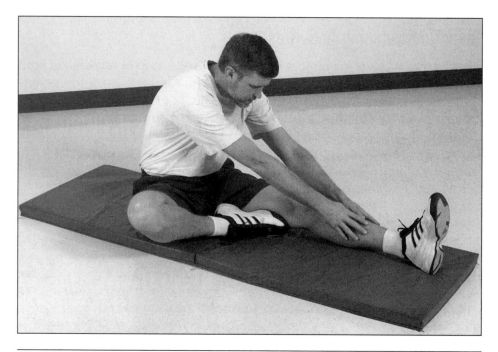

Figure 5.7 Sitting hamstring stretch.

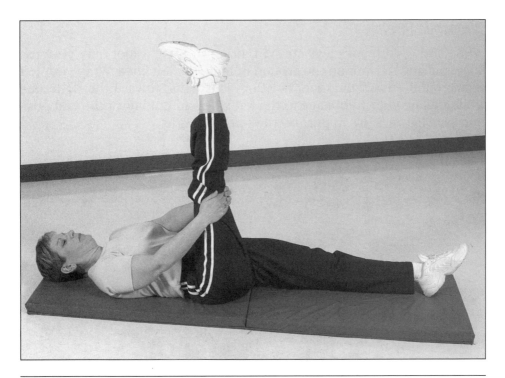

Figure 5.8 Lying hamstring stretch.

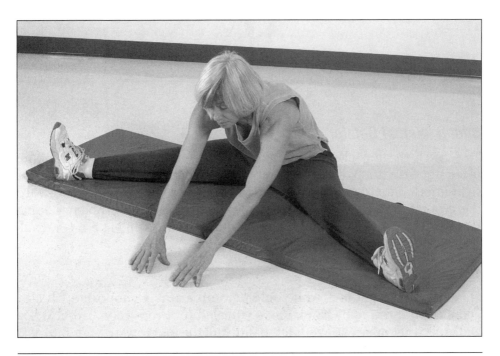

Figure 5.9 Groin stretch.

Piriformis Stretch

While sitting with your legs straight, bring your right foot over your left knee, placing the foot on the ground outside the left knee. Wrap your left arm around your right knee, twisting your trunk toward the right side while pulling your right knee to the left side and holding at the end position (see figure 5.10). Repeat on the opposite side.

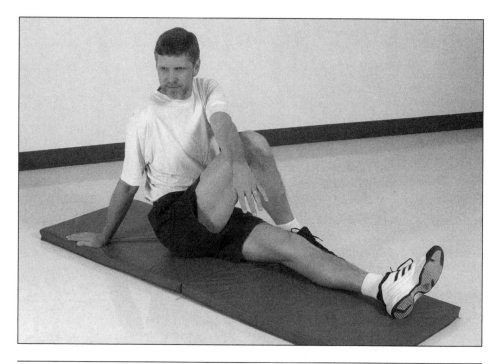

Figure 5.10 Piriformis stretch.

Sitting Internal Rotator Stretch

To stretch the muscles that rotate your hip in the opposite direction, place your right ankle on your left thigh, just above the knee. Let your right knee come toward the ground, and apply a gentle pressure toward the ground. Repeat with the opposite leg. If you have problems doing this exercise on the ground, it can be done while sitting in a chair, as illustrated in figure 5.11.

Hip Flexor Stretch

Stand on your right foot while holding onto a stable support, such as a counter, with the right hand. Raise your left foot toward your buttocks, and grab your ankle with your left hand. Pull the foot toward your buttock, while pressing your hip forward (see figure 5.12). Repeat this stretch with the opposite leg.

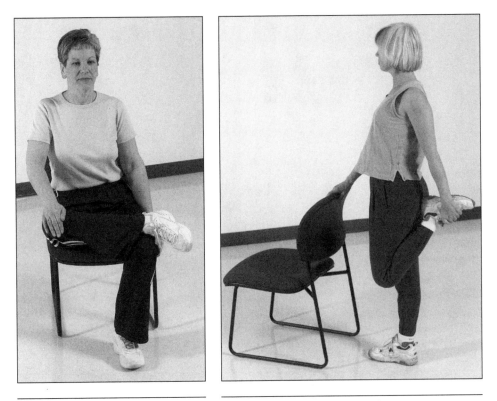

Figure 5.11 Sitting internal rotator stretch.

Figure 5.12 Hip flexor stretch.

Calf Stretches

Face a wall or counter and place your hands on it for support. Bring one leg back about 2 to 3 feet, with the foot flat on the ground and pointed straight forward. Bring your weight forward over the front leg, keeping the knee of the back leg straight and your back heel flat on the ground (see figure 5.13a). This exercise will stretch the gastrocnemius. To stretch the soleus muscle, bend the back knee, still keeping your foot flat on the ground (see figure 5.13b). Repeat this sequence with the opposite leg.

The upper body muscles that normally need stretching are the anterior shoulder and the internal rotator muscles. These stretches are usually done while standing, and most of them use a wall, doorway, or counter to assist with the stretch. Each exercise stretches the muscles in a slightly different way. I do not recommend a specific order—find the order that you prefer for whichever muscles are tight.

Pectoral Stretch

You can do this stretch standing in a doorway or in a corner. Raise both arms to just below shoulder height, with elbows bent to 90 degrees and

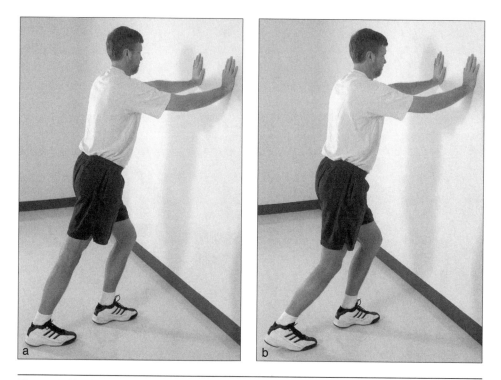

Figure 5.13   Calf stretches for (a) the gastrocnemius and (b) the soleus.

palms facing forward. If you use a doorway, place your hands on the door-jambs and lean your trunk forward slightly (see figure 5.14). In a corner, place a hand on each wall and lean into the corner. If you do not have a doorway or corner, bring both hands behind your head and move your elbows back until you feel a stretch in your chest.

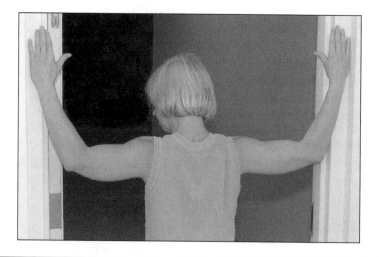

Figure 5.14   Pectoral stretch.

Upper Pectoral Stretch

This movement is easiest to do using a counter or dresser. Face the counter and place your hands on it. Step back until you are several feet away from the counter and your hips bend at a 90-degree angle. Allow your trunk weight to drop further, stretching the front of your shoulders gently (see figure 5.15).

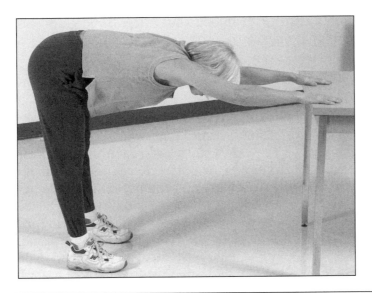

Figure 5.15   Upper pectoral stretch.

Rotator Stretch

While standing in a doorway, position yourself so that your right elbow is at your side, with your right hand holding the doorjamb. Turn your trunk gently toward the left, keeping the elbow and hand in position (see figure 5.16). Repeat this movement with your left shoulder.

Here is a final word about stretching and technique. Regardless of the technique that is used, proper body position is vital to the result. A simple alteration in your pelvic position can diminish the resultant change in hamstring flexibility. Keep your trunk as upright as possible for all hip stretches, letting the motion come from your hip and not from your low back. Point your

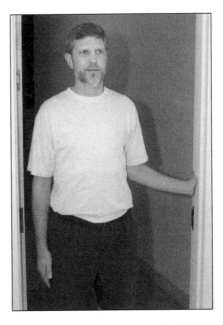

Figure 5.16   Rotator stretch.

knees and toes straight ahead, and do not rotate your hips unless the instructions direct you to do so.

Movements to Avoid

Some positions and activities may actually cause damage and are therefore not recommended. The specific movements may vary according to your particular arthritic problems, but a few basic guidelines on types of movements that may cause problems can help you decide whether to do a specific activity.

Overstretching

The first rule is that one should never overstretch (that is, take the muscle past its normal range of motion). Although athletes may be able to tolerate overstretching when they are young, most arthritic joints already have some instability present, and overstretching the surrounding muscles may increase both the instability and the potential for damage. In addition, muscle tissues that are inflamed during arthritic flare-ups are more prone to damage. You may need to decrease the intensity of a stretch as well as the number of repetitions until your arthritis has calmed down. Areas that I have seen people overstretch include the neck, back, and shoulders.

Signs of Overstretching

▷ Extreme motions

▷ Pain during a stretch

▷ Rapid, uncontrolled stretches

▷ Sharp, shooting pains or muscle cramps

Extreme Joint Motions

Yoga is an example of an activity that may use extreme joint ranges and that you must modify to avoid stressing your joints. Yoga is an excellent activity that is often used for flexibility; however, I believe that some of the movements put you at risk for further joint damage. An example is the "plough" position, illustrated in figure 5.17. This position puts the neck in extreme flexion, which can stress joints that are already at risk because of your arthritis. It would be impossible to identify every position you should avoid, especially as it depends on your individual joint involvement. You need to decide whether a movement is extreme and whether you can modify it or should avoid it altogether.

Movement That Increases Pain

The second guideline is that the movement should not increase your pain. Although arthritis is by definition painful, the pain should not worsen during an exercise. Increased pain can have several causes, including a

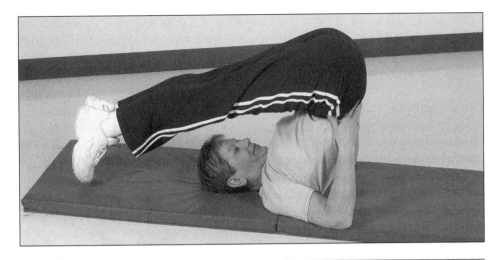

Figure 5.17 The plough position.

too rapid motion, overstretching, improper technique, and the severity of your disease. If your joint disease is exceptionally severe, you may need to attempt only part of the range for the initial program, and you may want to unload the joint (decrease the compressive forces acting on the joint). Unloading the joint can be accomplished by performing the activities in the water or by using gentle distraction, such as a pulley, to assist with the motion. During flare-ups you may need to decrease the number of repetitions of range of motion exercises.

Personalizing Your Program

Each person has specific needs for flexibility, just as for a total program and for each of its components. Design this component of your program based on the cardiovascular and strength activities you plan to do and on your personal flexibility problems. I run several days a week and do resistance work two days a week. Running tends to tighten the hamstrings, quadriceps, and calf muscles, so I know they need attention in my regular stretching routine. Because of previous injuries and stiffness, I stretch these muscles everyday, even if I am not exercising. The only areas of my upper body that have limited flexibility are my anterior shoulders, quite a common problem for those of us who work at a desk a lot. These areas I stretch twice a week when doing resistance work, and I do more generalized range of motion activities for my shoulders every day.

One of the keys to personalizing a flexibility program is to creatively combine stretching and flexibility activities to suit your needs. I have identified only a few stretches and range of motion activities; there are entire texts devoted to these topics. However, with the principles that I have discussed, you can design a range of motion or stretching routine to meet your specific need.

Earlier in the book, I used the example of a gentleman who wanted to improve his flexibility for golf. If you analyze a golf swing, you can see that you need hip, trunk, and shoulder flexibility to produce a good, complete swing. I would start by having him stretch daily. Once he had obtained optimal range of motion, he could concentrate on range of motion activities to maintain his movement. If he wanted to individualize the stretching even more, rather than use basic stretches such as those shown in this chapter, he could do stretches that simulate the golf motion required. For example, when you hit a golf ball, you shift your weight from one leg to the other while rotating your trunk. He could manage this combination, holding the position at the end of each major movement. Many golfers do a modification of these movements, holding the golf club in both hands and twisting from side to side.

In this chapter I have discussed the primary principles of flexibility exercise and ways to achieve increased range of motion. I have presented some simple range of motion activities that will help decrease stiffness and joint pain. In addition, I have described some basic stretches for use with tight muscles or joints that may lack full range. At this point all of the components of a traditional exercise program have been presented, and you have the tools to design a good fitness program. However, not everyone likes to exercise alone, and one alternative I have not yet addressed is exercise classes. In chapter 6, I will discuss several different types of exercise classes and the pros and cons of each. Many people I work with like to alternate doing a traditional exercise program with participating in an exercise class.

ACTION PLAN:
PURSUING FLEXIBILITY

☐ Be aware of necessary preparations for a flexibility program:

- How will you deal with muscle stiffness due to temperature?
- Is your muscle strength balanced around a joint?

☐ Assess your current condition or level of flexibility and decide which type of activity to engage in (such as static stretching and active range of motion).

☐ Choose stretches and build your program to be compatible with your aerobic and strength activities and your personal flexibility needs (strengths and weaknesses).

☐ Be aware of the things to avoid in order to ensure safety in stretching.

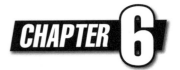

EXPLORING ALTERNATIVE EXERCISE PROGRAMS

Many people do not like to exercise alone, and exercising with a group can be an excellent support mechanism. When a friend of my mother was diagnosed with rheumatoid arthritis, she joined an aquatic exercise class for people with arthritis. The class is like a support group for her, and with regular exercise and medications, she has been able to resume some of the activities that she had given up before her diagnosis. Others have told me that they enjoy classes because they are surrounded by peers and because the classes are designed with the specific problems of arthritis patients in mind.

Exercise classes can have several pros and cons, depending on the specific class that you are considering. The benefit of exercising with people who have problems similar to yours is substantial. A class designed for people with arthritis uses movements and activities that are more suited to stiff joints and limited ranges of motion. Most such classes use low-impact activities with lessened intensity and include more warm-up and cool-down activities in the session. Psychologically, it can build up your self-esteem to feel you are part of a group.

On the other hand, if you decide to join an exercise class that is designed for a younger, fitter clientele, you may find it does not fit your needs. Although being around young, vibrant people can be invigorating, it can also be discouraging if you cannot keep up with the pace of a class or if you are a person who compares yourself to those around you. Such frustration can lead to discontinuing exercise altogether rather than modifying the activity. Furthermore, some exercise classes include activities that put arthritic joints under excessive stress, potentially increasing pain and stiffness.

If you prefer to exercise in a group, look for classes designed for people with arthritis or classes with low-impact activities. Many hospitals and facilities offer health and fitness classes for specific groups, such as arthritis patients. Qualified instructors who are educated about special needs related to arthritis usually teach their classes. The Arthritis Foundation has developed community-based programs offered nationwide through the YMCA and other facilities.

Determine whether the facility is easily accessible to you and whether the class hours suit your schedule. I suggest going in and observing a session before joining a class; in this way you can evaluate the level of intensity, the types of movements related to your needs, and even the kind of music used in the class. Pay close attention to how the instructor interacts with the participants; keep away from a class in which the instructor comes across like a drill sergeant. A good instructor should check on individuals occasionally, slowing some down and speeding others up. I like instructors who include some education at the beginning of a course—it shows they are interested in meeting your needs.

Questions to Consider When Choosing an Exercise Class

▷ How many people are in the class?

▷ Is the location convenient and comfortable?

▷ Is the class designed for people with arthritis? If not, can I alter the activities to meet my needs?

▷ Does the class include a warm-up and a cool-down?

▷ What is the average fitness level of the participants, and does it match mine?

▷ Is the instructor well qualified, and how does he or she interact with the class?

▷ Is the atmosphere one that I would enjoy? For example, if there is music, does it sound like something I would like, or is it too loud?

▷ Are there other classes at other times that I can attend, if I want to make up missed classes?

▷ Is the staff prepared to deal with minor and major emergencies? Are they certified in CPR or first aid?

You can consider several types of group classes, each with potential benefits. Most classes try to include each component of fitness in the activities. The cardiovascular conditioning benefits may not be as substantial as an equally long session of pure aerobic exercise, but you get the advantage of a well-rounded program. The most common types of classes are aerobics (both on land and in water), tai chi, and yoga classes. Other group classes can be beneficial, but these are the most common. Evaluate the one you are considering using the general guidelines provided here.

Aerobics Classes

Aerobics classes were given their name many years ago, when the concept of a class conducted with music was first introduced. I have divided such classes into land and aquatic classes, although one could also divide them according to the emphasis, intensity, or purpose of the class. For example, "spinning" is a new type of class that has developed within the last few years. Spinning classes are basically group aerobic classes that use stationary cycles as the workout mode. Each of the various types of land and aquatic classes also emphasize particular elements.

Land Classes

The benefits of participating in aerobics derive from the focus of the class and the frequency of your participation. A class that meets only once a week has limited health benefits, although it might be fun as a change of pace from a more traditional exercise regimen. Look for a class that meets at least three days per week in order to reap any fitness gains. Studies have shown that aerobics participation reduces pain and improves lower-extremity function, strength, walking speed or distance, and aerobic power, which is an estimate of aerobic endurance from a short activity (Perlman et al. 1990; Noreau et al. 1995). Most of these studies also found decreased depression after completion of a class. They have identified cardiovascular benefits only when the frequency is at least three times per week and the intensity is appropriate (as identified in chapter 3—50 to 85 percent of HRR).

What to Look For in a Class

As stated earlier, look for an aerobics class that either is intended for individuals with arthritis or uses only low-impact activities. A low-impact class means that there is not a lot of bouncing and jumping, both of which can be very stressful to your joints. Low-impact classes also have fewer injuries associated with them than do high-impact classes (Janis 1990).

The general fitness benefits of a well-designed aerobics class are determined by its components, although the strengthening benefits are limited. The class should have a warm-up period during which the activity is slowly increased, a period devoted to cardiovascular activity (rhythmic activity using larger muscle groups), and a cool-down period. In addition, most will have some calisthenic activity that is designed to tone the muscles. The resistance is usually your limb or body weight, so the focus is on building muscular endurance.

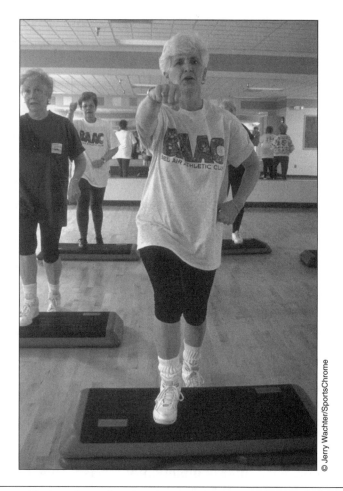

© Jerry Wachter/SportsChrome

Aerobics classes offer benefits such as low-impact motion and activities for all of the fitness components.

A good instructor is essential. Find out the instructor's qualifications and experience. This is not to say that a new instructor cannot be good, but make sure that he understands the principles of exercise and knows how to help people with activity adjustments. Several groups offer certification, which ensures at least a basic level of knowledge on the instructor's part. The Arthritis Foundation programs provide instructor training that covers not only exercise principles but also information specific to arthritis.

In the 1980s the Arthritis Foundation introduced a program called PACE (People with Arthritis Can Exercise), which is offered nationwide. If you have one of these programs in your community, I highly recommend it. The classes are designed for people with arthritis, and they have a proven record of accomplishment. They provide education on body mechanics, joint protection, and the basic principles of exercise. The program offers two levels of instruction, a basic and an advanced level, which should meet the needs of most participants. When in doubt, start with the basic class to lower the risk of an overuse injury from starting at too high a level.

Basic Requirements

Look for a class that includes the normal components of exercise identified earlier—warm-up, cardiovascular exercise, strength and flexibility activities, and a cool-down. The length of a class is usually 45 to 60 minutes. A good 60-minute class contains at least 10 minutes of warm-up activity, 15 to 20 minutes of large movement aerobics, and 10 minutes of cool-down. The warm-up and cool-down may incorporate range of motion and stretching activities. The rest of the time is usually devoted to muscular conditioning exercises.

Estimate your own target heart rate, as shown in chapter 3. Use this rate to monitor your exercise intensity. I often see people working at too high a level, because they are trying to keep up with the instructor and others around them. Remember, the instructor has been doing this routine for a while and is probably at a different fitness level than you are. If your limbs feel extremely heavy or experience a burning sensation, then you are working more anaerobically than aerobically. In other words, you are producing lactic acid because you are working at too high an intensity, and you need to decrease it. Use the talk test—you should not be breathing so heavily that you cannot respond to a simple question with a short phrase. On the other hand, if you are able to chat with someone, then you are not working hard enough. Again, refer to your target heart rate to assess your intensity.

You may need to modify some of the activities based on your limitations. For example, if you have arthritis in your shoulders, perform only the upper body activities that do not cause increased pain. If the instructor tells the class to do a rapid arm movement overhead, slow down the movement and do it at shoulder level. With lower-extremity arthritis, you may find that you cannot do some of the activities that require lots of rotation at the hip or extreme hip and knee flexion. Usually you can do such motions through a shorter range.

I recommend that you participate in an aerobics class no more than three days per week. The rate of overuse injuries increases with increased frequency of participation in traditional aerobics classes, so limiting the frequency to three days per week should also limit the potential for injury (Rothenberger, Chang, and Cable 1988; Janis 1990). On the alternate days, you can carry out a more traditional cardiovascular program, such as walking, or perhaps a different kind of activity. Not only will your chance of injury decrease, but the varied routine may also help you stick with your program.

As with walking or jogging, you need to make sure that you have good shoes. The types of shoes that are appropriate for jogging are not the same as the ones you need for an aerobics class. Your shoes should have more support in the forefoot as well as adequate cushioning. These shoes may be called "cross-trainers" or something similar. In chapter 7, I discuss what to look for in shoes in greater detail. Usually you do not need special clothing as long as what you wear is comfortable and absorbent.

Water Aerobics

Exercise in the water has some unique benefits compared to other programs. The buoyancy of the water reduces the amount of body weight placing stress on joints, and the warmth of the water can lessen muscle stiffness. Movements tend to be less vigorous in a water class, a quality that also contributes to decreased joint stress. Participating in water aerobics classes with appropriate frequency, duration, and intensity can improve your aerobic and functional capacity and decrease pain (Minor et al. 1989; Sanford-Smith, MacKay-Lyons, and Nunes-Clement 1998). Many people tell me that they enjoy and stick with an aquatic class because "it feels great in the water." One woman reports that she likes aquatic classes in the winter when she cannot get outside as easily. Incorporating an aquatic class into your regimen may be especially beneficial if you have multiple joint involvements, rheumatoid arthritis, or more advanced arthritis.

What to Look For in a Class

As with the land aerobics classes, look for classes specifically designed for people with arthritis. The Arthritis Foundation and the YMCA have developed an aquatic program for people with arthritis that is available nationwide. These classes have been proven effective; they are currently offered at two levels. The focus of the aquatic program is range of motion improvement and muscle strengthening, with an optional segment for building endurance (classes with the endurance segment are longer). If you are considering an aquatic class not designed for persons with arthritis, go in and watch a class. Look for a class that is not too large so that participants can move freely without bumping into one another. An aquatic class, like a land class, should begin with a warm-up period, include both upper- and lower-extremity activities, and end with a cool-down segment. The pace should be brisk and the activities varied.

As with land classes, the Arthritis Foundation/YMCA program provides training to their instructors. Therefore, you know that your teacher has the necessary education about the exercise requirements and special needs of arthritic people. If you check out other programs, look for an instructor who has experience in aquatic exercise and who knows how to adapt movements to individual needs. Any instructor should have basic Red Cross or YMCA lifesaving certification as well as instructor certification. A good teacher includes an education segment, usually before anyone gets into the water, and helps you individualize movements for your capabilities.

Two environmental factors to consider are the temperature and depth of the water. Usually classes designed for people with arthritis have addressed these issues, but it helps to know what to look for. Water temperature should be between 84 and 92 degrees Fahrenheit, slightly warmer than pools that are used primarily for lap swimming. Exercises should take place in water that ranges from mid-chest to shoulder level in depth. The deeper the water, the lower the stress (from gravity) placed on joints in your lower extremities. If you are standing in water that reaches the lower end of your sternum, your body is unloaded by approximately 75 percent.

Basic Requirements

The basic requirements of a program in the water are the same as for a land program—warm-up segment, all three fitness components, and a cool-down period—combined in a class of 45 to 60 minutes. Special water exercise equipment is available to provide an effective resistance component to your program. These devices increase resistance either by enlarging the surface area that pushes against the water, as a hand paddle does, or by increasing the buoyancy of a limb. When you try to push a buoyant object under the water, there is greater resistance to your motion. Although there is some resistance to any motion through the water, such devices can greatly enhance an aquatic exercise class. A good aquatics instructor should explain and demonstrate each new activity before you execute the movement, especially when using equipment such as I have described.

You can safely participate in a water aerobics class five days per week, although you might find that three days per week is enough. Again, try alternating the type of program you do on different days, to give variety to your routine. An important difference between the basic requirements of aquatic programs and land programs is the estimation of work intensity. Your heart rate decreases simply by getting into the water; thus, heart rate may not accurately reflect the true intensity at which you are working. You can try using the same target heart rate you use for land, but you may find that you do not feel as if you are working at as high a level. If necessary, use rating of perceived exertion to evaluate and modify your intensity.

One piece of clothing that you might not think about for an aquatic class is shoes. Because you exercise while standing on the bottom of the pool, your feet can become sore. Get a pair of water shoes—padded slippers with nonskid soles that reduce foot discomfort and lower the chance of slipping.

Tai Chi

You may have heard of tai chi but have thought that it is not appropriate for you, especially with your arthritis. Although it originated in the martial arts, several forms of tai chi have been modified to emphasize health benefits. Tai chi focuses on slow, controlled movements throughout a complete range of motion, with minimal impact on the lower extremities. The benefits of tai chi include improved balance and flexibility, some cardiovascular enhancement, and the psychological benefits typically reported with exercise (Matsuda 2003; Young et al. 1999; Lan et al. 1998). Both people who have osteoarthritis and those who have rheumatoid arthritis have used tai chi effectively (Kirstein, Dietz, and Hwang 1991; Lumsden, Baccala, and Martire 1998). Arthritis patients report that the activity does not aggravate their arthritis and helps decrease their stiffness and fatigue.

A few years ago some of my students worked with a local senior center, comparing the benefits of different types of group activities. Those that did tai chi demonstrated the best adherence to their programs. They reported that they enjoyed the classes immensely, because the movements were easy to follow and because they were not afraid of hurting themselves (in contrast to some participants in the other activities). Numerous articles cite this type of anecdotal evidence, demonstrating that new activities such as tai chi are worth a try.

What to Look For in a Class

Some information about the history of tai chi, as well as its forms and principles, helps one know what to look for in a class. Tai chi chuan originated in China as a martial art. As with many Eastern practices, it strives to balance the mind and the body by using a blend of focused movement and meditation. The word "chuan" is not used with some of the newer forms, since the emphasis on the combative aspects of the discipline has been removed. Different forms (styles) of tai chi use different numbers of moves, ranging from 9 to 108; the most common form uses 24 moves. Five principles serve as the guide for the forms. These principles include the separation of yin and yang (opposing energy), keeping the body upright, the waist is the commander, the body is relaxed and movement is flowing and yielding, and attention to present (focus on the movement) (Matsuda 2002).

For a specialized class such as tai chi, one of the first things I look at is the instructor's qualifications. A good instructor has several years of experience in this martial art. I investigated taking a class a few years ago, but decided not to when I found that the "instructor" had only taken one class before deciding to teach it. I would have gotten a more professional training by renting a videotape! A good instructor incorporates education into the class and circulates among class members to correct body postures or refine movements. A smaller class is preferable at the beginning levels, since it allows more individualized attention from the instructor. The class should identify its level so that a beginner is not struggling to keep up with those who have been practicing tai chi for years. Many beginning classes focus on shorter routines that use basic movements or techniques.

Basic Requirements

The benefits of tai chi are greatest in the areas of flexibility and lower-extremity strength. Although you can derive some cardiovascular benefits from tai chi, it does not stimulate the cardiovascular system optimally. To develop a well-balanced exercise program, I suggest doing a cardiovascular exercise program on alternating days with a tai chi class. A well-designed class starts with posture and breathing activities, along with some simple weight shifts and waist turns. After a warm-up period of 15 or more minutes, it progresses to whole body techniques combined with arm and hand movements. A good introductory class introduces only a few forms each session and adds one or two new moves each week. The movements are slow and controlled, flowing from one position to another.

As in other classes, you may need to modify movements because of your arthritis. A videotape on tai chi that I viewed demonstrates movements, such as deep knee bends, that could easily aggravate knee and hip pain. From what I have observed, the primary modifications you may need to make are in the ranges of the movements, but not in speed or repetitions. Other modifications that you may need to make include limiting single stance time and decreasing internal rotation at the hip. As with any exercise, adjust the move based on your pain and your joint limitations. Some classes are designed for people of limited ability and use grab bars or other methods of support to promote safety.

The recommended attire for a tai chi class includes loose, comfortable clothing and soft-soled shoes. If your class is indoors (in warmer climates these classes may be offered outdoors), you can wear a nonskid shoe with thinner soles. For outdoor classes, a walking or tennis shoe gives you better support on uneven ground.

Tai Chi Variations

Several groups have taken the traditional practice of tai chi and modified it to use for health purposes. A range of motion dance program was developed using the principles of tai chi, which has been further adapted for people with various disabilities (Harlowe and Yu 1997). Elderly persons have used a modification that employs nine movements to help reduce falls. Such programs are not traditional tai chi, but you may find that one of them meets your needs for a group class with low-impact activity.

Yoga

Yoga is another nontraditional exercise that has potential benefits for people with arthritis. As with tai chi, its original purpose is not exercise, but in this case, a means of achieving self-understanding. The National Coalition for Complimentary and Alternative Medicine has classified yoga as a "mind-body" therapy because of its emphasis on physical and mental integration. The most common form in the United States is hatha yoga, which focuses on postures and breathing control. Yoga may be helpful in developing and maintaining flexibility, coordination, muscle tone, and balance. Participation in yoga appears to yield specific physical benefits (such as lower blood pressure and cholesterol) as well as improved exercise tolerance (Austin and Laeng 2003). The research demonstrates that benefits for people with arthritis are limited, but promising. These benefits include decreased pain and improved range of motion (Garfinkel et al. 1994). Some people swear by yoga for its effect on improving and maintaining flexibility, as well as for its meditative properties.

What to Look For in a Class

As with tai chi, some information about the history and types of yoga may be helpful in evaluating a class. Yoga started in India more than 2000 years ago, and numerous styles have evolved through the years. The practice of yoga is a meditative one, intended to bring one to a deeper understanding of the universe and of truth, although it has developed a greater focus on physical aspects (Austin and Laeng 2003).

Hatha yoga, as already noted, is one of the most common forms practiced on the North American continent. Even within this form, there are many styles with slightly different focuses. In general, there are eight philosophical principles, called ashtangas, which guide yoga practice. Two of these, asana and pranayama, serve as the basis of hatha yoga; they guide physical postures and breathing patterns, although the other principles are also used. Techniques and principles are supposed to have specific benefits related to different physiological systems. For example, some of the pranayama techniques are supposed to help the respiratory system through back extension coordinated with breathing patterns. A few yoga styles have been developed for therapeutic purposes and use modified positions and some equipment.

As when considering any other class, you should ask a few questions:

1. What is the focus of this particular class and for whom is it designed?
2. What are the instructor's credentials?
3. Does the instructor individualize physical postures?
4. Are equipment adaptations available if necessary?

You may find that a class designed for older or arthritic people is preferable, at least to start with. The postures are less likely to be extreme and some adaptations using equipment are usually included. Two modifications that I think are vital are mats and some sort of railing or stable support device. Doing some of the postures on a hard floor can aggravate stiffness and pain. A grab bar can increase safety when performing challenging one-legged standing postures.

The better instructors have a few years of experience, both with yoga and with various physical limitations. Each style of yoga has its own set of teacher certification standards, which can be frustrating if you are trying to find out about your instructor's credentials. One effort to address this problem has been the creation of the Yoga Alliance Registry, which identifies minimum standards and includes all styles. I have supplied contact information for the registry in the resources section at the end of the book.

Basic Requirements

Because yoga is not primarily focused on exercise, it is difficult to determine what basic requirements a class should meet. The primary benefits, as already noted, are flexibility, balance, and some muscle tone. Therefore, you can practice yoga on a daily basis to meet the flexibility component of your training. If you are looking for a well-balanced exercise program, include another type of activity to meet your cardiovascular and strength-training needs.

The duration of yoga classes varies, but the most common community-based programs seem to last between 40 and 60 minutes. Classes usually begin with a basic posture, focusing on breathing, alignment, and body awareness. Postures progress from simple to more difficult and attempt to use a variety of motions. The most common postures involve standing on one leg or both legs, bending forward and backward, sitting, and twisting. Most yoga sessions finish with relaxation postures (Austin and Laeng 2003).

You may need to modify or eliminate some of the more than one hundred postures, for safety reasons. Although no formal contraindications exist for yoga, I believe that you should avoid some postures or at least approach them with caution. I put these postures into two broad classes: those that put unusual stresses on a joint and those that may put stress on a system, such as the cardiovascular system. Some postures may do both. The chapter on flexibility includes an illustration of a posture that could potentially do both. The plough position requires you to lie on the ground and bring your feet over your head, with your legs straight, until your feet touch the ground behind your head. If you have arthritis in your neck, this pose could injure those joints. If you have cardiovascular disease, such as high blood pressure or atherosclerosis (narrowing of the arteries), this position might also stress your system; you may want to limit inverted poses because of the potential effect on blood flow.

Clothing for yoga should be comfortable and nonrestricting. It can be loose and somewhat baggy, such as shorts and a T-shirt or stretchy exercise wear. Whatever you wear, you need to be able to move freely without getting caught in excess folds. One yoga teacher I talked to likes to have everyone barefoot. Being barefoot may not be comfortable if you have arthritis in your feet; a lightweight athletic shoe may be more appropriate. Your shoe should have a nonskid sole and give you adequate support and comfort.

Personalizing Your Program

For each type of class, I have identified ways in which you may need to adjust the activity to accommodate your joint restrictions or personal needs. These methods include slowing down to decrease the cardiovascular intensity; eliminating activities that you cannot do because of joint limitations or pain; and decreasing extreme motions, especially knee and hip flexion. Beyond such adjustments in motion or intensity, classes are not set up for personalization. These types of classes can be used, however, to personalize your entire exercise regimen.

Most classes work best when done two to three days per week, a schedule that allows you to put a different emphasis into your daily program on the remaining days. None of these classes offers optimal cardiovascular or strength conditioning, so I suggest setting up a program that emphasizes these elements at least two days of the week, alternating with the group classes. Another option is to view a group class as an adjunct to your normal program. For example, the university recreation center near me offers tai chi each semester, one day per week. Once a week is not enough to gain any significant benefits, but I can do it as a way to add a group activity into my program. My base exercise regimen can take place five days a week, with the typical components; on the sixth day, I can do tai chi.

Group classes are a pleasant way to incorporate a social aspect into your program, and the variety may help improve adherence to your pro-

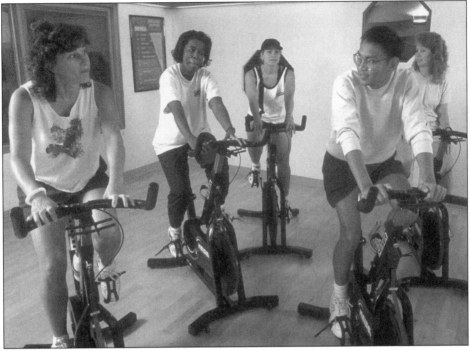

Many people enjoy the social setting a group class provides.

gram. Repeatedly I hear how people like the support they get from being with a group, especially when the group has similar health concerns, such as arthritis. If you are an outgoing person, consider joining a class as an adjunct to your program—it may greatly increase your enjoyment of your exercise routine.

In this chapter I have discussed various types of exercise classes, including aerobics on land and in the water, tai chi, and yoga. You may come across other types of classes that you wish to consider. Always observe the class and the types of movements it employs first. I have discussed the requirements for each component of fitness, so you can analyze the activities and determine whether the class meets any of these requirements and whether it uses movements that you might find stressful to an arthritic joint.

I have now dealt with most forms of exercise, but it is also necessary to address joint protection. Joint protection is critical for anyone participating in exercise, but especially for people with arthritis. Arthritis is a progressive disease; although exercise does not speed up joint deterioration, it also does not slow it. Some activities put extra stress on joints, which proper techniques and joint protection devices can ease. The next chapter identifies joint protection strategies.

ACTION PLAN:
CONSIDERING ALTERNATIVE EXERCISE OPTIONS

☐ Find out what types of groups or classes are available in your area.

☐ Visit classes and answer the questions listed at the beginning of the chapter.

☐ Choose a class, and make the necessary preparations:

- Measure your heart rate.
- Secure necessary equipment (shoes, clothing, and so forth).
- Check out location conditions such as pool temperature, etc.

☐ Adjust the activity according to your joint restrictions or painful areas.

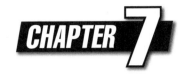

CHAPTER 7

PROTECTING YOUR JOINTS

Joint protection matters for everyone with arthritis, even if one is in the early stages of arthritis and does not have noticeable joint instability. Exercise does not normally accelerate the progression of arthritis, but some activities can put additional stresses on joints. Compromised tissues do not respond to these forces in the same manner that healthy tissues do. Less than optimal tissue response combined with excessive joint stress can lead to injury; thus, one must reduce any unusual stresses that might put pressure on a joint.

We have already discussed two primary ways to protect your joints—strengthening the surrounding tissues and maintaining proper flexibility. Even with such measures, poor biomechanics magnify the stress transmitted to a joint. A significant relationship exists between poor alignment of the knee joint and the progression of osteoarthritis, regardless of age, sex, or body weight (Sharma et al. 2001). You can protect your joints by using correct posture and appropriate equipment, and by controlling weight, eating properly, and taking beneficial supplements. Protecting your joints allows you to participate in the activities you enjoy for a longer time and with greater comfort.

Posture

Posture has an important relationship to exercise that is often overlooked. As I noted previously, improper habitual resting posture can affect muscular flexibility and the resultant joint mechanics. Exercise is a critical means of correcting muscle imbalance and expanding the available motion around a joint, but it is only part of the answer. Consider that your waking day lasts at least 12 hours and exercise takes up only about 1 hour, leaving 11 hours of activities that affect your resting posture. When one was admonished to sit or stand up straight while growing up, it was for valid reasons. Not only does a person look better, but proper posture is vital to good health. Poor posture is connected to back and neck pain, shoulder dysfunction, and hip and knee pain (Kendall, McCreary, and Provance 1993).

Often people who seek treatment for knee pain are actually suffering pain referred from their backs. They may have arthritis in their knees as well, but they may have two sources of pain rather than one. Whenever I visited my grandmother, she would ask me what to do for her hip. She had been told the hip was arthritic, and she had pain along that thigh. My grandmother was an avid walker, and this pain was starting to interfere with her walking. With a few simple tests, I determined that the pain was not coming from her hip. She did have arthritis in her hip but could move her hip through almost its complete range without pain, while back movements reproduced and exacerbated her pain. A visit to a specialist confirmed that her back was the source of her pain. Unfortunately, at 95 years old, her back joints also had significant deterioration, which sitting did not help. She was able to keep walking, but with decreased frequency.

The classic test of good standing posture is if a vertical line can pass through the ear, the tip of the shoulder, the middle of the hip, the back of the knee, and the front of the ankle (see figure 7.1). It is called the line of gravity and represents an equal distribution of forces behind and in front of the major joints. Simply described, proper posture is standing tall with your spine in neutral, your chest lifted and your head and shoulders pulled back over the trunk. Most people have a slightly slumped posture—pelvis tilted forward, shoulders rounded, and head jutting out in front.

A good way to check your standing posture is by using a wall. Stand with your back to the wall and your heels against it (or within a few inches of it). With proper standing posture, you should have your buttocks, shoulder blades, and the back of your head touching the wall; your face looks straight ahead, without tilting up or down. This position feels unnatural if you have not had good posture for a while, but it becomes easier to maintain with practice. Work at holding this posture while walking as well. Good standing posture actually uses less energy because your muscles do not have to exert extra force against gravity.

Poor sitting posture has become more of a problem as people spend more time working at desks and computers. In addition, many of the chairs and sofas do not adequately support the lower back. Proper sitting posture is similar to standing posture for the trunk; a vertical line should pass through the middle of the ear, tip of the shoulder and middle of the hip.

A common improper sitting posture is a slumped position, with the lower back rounded and shoulders and head slouched forward. Correcting your sitting posture may require you to support your lower back and adjust your position relative to the equipment you are using. For example, most sofas are soft and do not support the back at all. A small pillow placed behind your lower back may shift you into a more upright

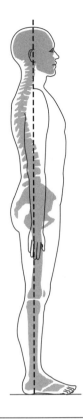

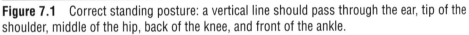

Figure 7.1 Correct standing posture: a vertical line should pass through the ear, tip of the shoulder, middle of the hip, back of the knee, and front of the ankle.

position. When driving, you should be close enough to the pedals that the seat completely supports your back and your head is directly over your trunk (close to or touching the headrest).

Good posture is habitual, and it may take time for you to acquire the habit. The potential benefits of working on your posture, however, are numerous. Proper body alignment is more efficient and is usually accompanied by good muscle balance and flexibility. Such posture reduces the stresses transmitted through your joints as well as any pain resulting from poor alignment.

Shoes

As discussed in the section on walking and running, good shoes are a vital component of your program. Appropriate footwear helps absorb landing forces and maintain joint alignment in your lower extremities during exercise. Specifics of the shoes vary slightly according to the activity for which they are designed. You can look for several features common to good exercise shoes, however, as noted in the sidebar on selecting footwear.

Selecting the Right Shoes

A good shoe has several qualities:

▷ A sole that provides shock absorption and cushioning

▷ Good arch support

▷ A roomy toe box that accommodates toe deformities

▷ A snug fit along the width of the shoe, especially in the heel counter. Walk or jog around the store in them—the heels should not slip.

▷ Removable inserts if you have orthotics. Take your orthotics with you so that you can try them in the shoe.

▷ Secure closure—lace-up is preferable, but Velcro may be necessary if you cannot manage laces due to arthritis in your hands

▷ A design appropriate for the activity you are doing. If you participate in several types of activities, consider cross-trainers, which are designed as multipurpose shoes.

Athletic shoes for different purposes differ in design, primarily in the sole (although some shoes can be used for multiple activities). Walking shoes, which you can usually wear throughout the day, have a flatter angle in the sole (heel to ball) and a smoother tread than a running shoe. Cross-trainers might be a good choice if you plan a regimen that includes a variety of training methods. Many people use these shoes for aerobics classes. They have a slightly steeper sole angle than a walking shoe and more padding under the ball of the foot than a running shoe. The cushioning in walking and cross-training shoes tends to be slightly firmer than in running shoes, because walking and aerobics do not generate the same landing impact as running. A shoe designed for tennis also has a thicker cushion, and the design of the sole enhances foot grip for the variety of moves that racquet sports require.

Golf shoes have a greater variety in basic design. Traditional golf shoes are similar to work-style shoes, with hard leather uppers and soles. Most of them do not support the arch well, making it important that you find one with enough room to put in inserts. Running shoe companies have started designing golf shoes that combine some of the requirements of a golf shoe with the comfort of a running or walking shoe. They tend to have a softer upper and sole, with more cushioning in the sole and arches. You can also obtain these shoes with permanent or removable soft spikes. Some of the women in my golf league who have arthritis tell me that the newer styles allow them to finish a game without the foot pain they used to have. Others have said that they golf in their walking shoes, eliminating the need for a special shoe.

Finally, keep in mind these tips for trying on exercise shoes. If you wear an orthotic, take it with you and try it in the shoe. This advice sounds like common sense, but several patients have told me they thought they could simply replace the manufactured insole with an orthotic and not affect the fit, only to find it made a major difference. Take or wear the type of socks you intend to wear with the shoes, since sock thickness also makes a difference in snugness.

Comfort is essential with any shoe, and you need to know that the shoes will remain comfortable during the activity for which you intend them. Wear the shoes for a while and move around in the store. Jog in place, simulate a golf swing, or simply walk back and forth several times. If they are not comfortable in the store, they will only feel worse when you are exercising for a longer period. A friend of mine finished the last few holes of a golf game barefoot, because she had severe pain and blisters from a new pair of shoes someone had given her, which she had not bothered to try on before playing. They were the right size and looked comfortable, so she did not think there would be a problem. Shoes are

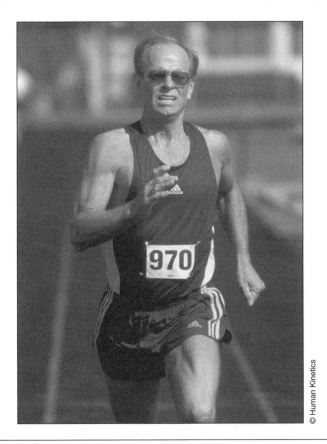

© Human Kinetics

Activities such as running can be hard on your joints, so put into practice techniques that protect your joints.

your most important piece of equipment for any land activity. Everyone has had an uncomfortable pair of shoes at some time; they can interfere with movement as well as comfort.

Once you have obtained good shoes, check them regularly for wear. A common problem that I see is people who wear shoes that no longer give them adequate support. You may need to replace your exercise shoes every three to six months, depending on their use. The more vigorous and regular your activity, the more quickly your shoes will break down.

Orthotics (Splints)

Orthotics, also known as splints, are devices that help align and support a joint in order to improve function and decrease pain. For patients with arthritis, numerous devices are available for the wrist, finger, knee, and foot. New materials and designs have decreased the bulkiness and improved the comfort and wear of orthotics. In addition, a wider variety of prefabricated orthotics, which are often less costly, are available on the market. The type of orthotic you need depends on the severity of your arthritis, degree of joint deformity, and the stress you put on that joint. If you have severe arthritis, pain, or deformity, your physician may prescribe a custom-made orthotic for you. In any case, if you plan on staying involved in an activity by using a splint, realize that you may have to modify your movements. Here I will focus on devices you can buy over the counter.

Wrist and Hand Splints

You may consider wrist or hand splints if you have arthritis in these joints and plan to engage in activities that stress them, such as golf, tennis, or weightlifting. Two general types of wrist splints are available—resting splints and work splints. For exercise you need a work (flexible) splint, since these allow more wrist movement. Most wrist splints stabilize by crossing over either the back or front of the wrist, with support around your forearm and some sort of closure around the palm of your hand. Because work splints allow more wrist movement, they provide less stability; therefore, you have to decide what you require.

If you have limited pain and sufficient stability, you might start with a simple elastic brace. This type of splint allows the greatest range of movement, while still giving some support to the wrist joint. With more pain and instability, check out a more rigid work splint. When you are trying on a splint, imitate the movements you use in your activity. Again, you will probably have to modify your motion slightly to perform the activity with a splint, and you are the only one who can determine whether the change will affect your performance more than you desire. My husband played in a golf tournament with a man who was wearing a wrist splint due to a severe arthritic flare-up. The man said that it did not detract from his game too much, whereas without the splint the pain affected his swing and concentration.

Finger Splints

Finger splints are indicated when you have boutonnière or swan-neck deformities. These splints are ring-type devices that help alignment of the joint, while preventing excessive movement in a specific direction. A splint for boutonnière deformity is designed to prevent flexion, while one for swan-neck deformity prevents hyperextension. Because most upper extremity activities require flexion of the fingers, the boutonnière splint has the greatest impact on activity. If you wear it on your dominant hand, you may need to do your exercise without it, and wear it the rest of the time. Doctors usually prescribe these splints for people who use their hands frequently.

Thumb splints have a slightly different design, except for the distal joint. Thumb splints can use a short hand base, or a longer base that extends up the forearm. A figure eight splint is a simple way to support the thumb joints while still allowing good movement. You may even have seen basketball players wearing a figure eight splint, since it is a common means of preventing excessive extension after a sprained thumb. Thus, they may also be useful for sports such as skiing, tennis, or even weight training. If you have significant instability, you will need a more rigid brace, with limited motion.

Knee Splints

The various types of knee splints differ in use, style, and complexity. The simplest knee brace is a neoprene sleeve. Neoprene sleeves are most useful if you have mild arthritis and your primary purpose is to reduce pain and swelling. This device does not provide alignment correction or structural support for the knee joint, although it may contribute some input to joint proprioception.

For realignment purposes, you can get several types of knee braces over the counter or custom fit by an orthotist. Custom fit braces are molded to your size and are usually of a higher quality; they are sometimes adjustable. Such braces are more expensive than over-the-counter braces, which have fewer options for adjusting fit. Realignment goals vary because they are based on your personal biomechanics. They include bicompartment, patellofemoral, and tibiofemoral realignment (Liu and Mirzayan 1995).

For some people, the goal of using a knee brace may be ligament protection. I recommend that you see someone qualified to determine which type of brace meets your needs and to fit you properly. Proper fit of a knee brace is essential, as an improper fit not only fails to realign the joint but also may lead to further joint damage. A gentleman I know used a brace for several years to reduce the pain in his knee during tennis, his preferred mode of exercise. Tennis puts lateral and torsional stresses on the knees, so a brace is a good way to reduce these stresses, which can damage arthritic knees.

Foot Orthotics

As with knee orthotics, foot orthotics are designed to realign the lower extremities, theoretically reducing the stress on the involved joints. Foot deformities develop over time in people with arthritis, leading clinicians to recommend orthotics as a method of preventing, or at least slowing, the deformation (Hanes 1996; Hillstrom et al. 2001a, 2001b). The most common problems that occur with arthritis are excess pronation, rolling in at the ankle, and loss of motion in some of the forefoot joints. As arthritis progresses, deformities can occur throughout the foot. Both the deformations and the abnormal movement can cause pain in the foot, ankle, knee, and even up into the hip.

There are three types of foot orthotics: flexible, semi-rigid, and rigid. If you have looked at shoe inserts in the pharmacy, you have probably looked at flexible or semi-rigid inserts. Over-the-counter, flexible inserts are the least costly, and they come in standard sizes and designs. The correction given is minimal, however, so use them only if you do not have too much misalignment and are primarily looking for additional shock absorption. If you have slight discomfort, you may try other insole modifications that are also less costly than custom orthotics. Inexpensive padding for the metatarsal (ball of the foot) or heel is available over the counter. Any modification should not cause pain, but help alleviate pain because of improved alignment. If the padding or insert increases existing pain or causes new pain, remove it immediately. Talk to your doctor before you try any drastic modifications.

Some manufacturers make semi-rigid orthotics that can be purchased over the counter; however, you need to know what sort of alignment problem you have. For more severe arthritic pain, deformity, and malalignment, see a healthcare provider who has experience designing orthotics for people with arthritis. Custom-made orthotics are more expensive, but they are tailored to your specific needs. They should provide better pain reduction and movement control when compared to a prefabricated insert.

Another source of foot pain that happens more frequently in middle-aged people and those with arthritis is plantar fasciitis. The hallmark of plantar fasciitis is extreme pain upon standing in the morning, greatest under the heel and arch. Initial treatment may include flexible heel cups that provide cushioning under the heel and help control pronation. With chronic pain, your physician or therapist may recommend a foot orthotic. I have had good results with some patients by using an aggressive approach during the initial symptoms. This multi-faceted approach includes frequent stretching of the calf muscles, self-massage of the sole of the foot, modification of shoes, and modified activity until the pain subsides. The shoe modification emphasizes good arch support and slight heel padding. If your symptoms do not resolve within a week or so, you need to see your physician or therapist.

Supplements

Think of joint protection as occurring from both the outside and the inside of your body. The external devices I have described can reduce pain and improve joint alignment so that you exercise with greater comfort. Companies advertise various supplements that they claim protect cartilage within the joints and reduce pain. Before discussing some of the supplements that research has recognized as having potential benefits, I will address some of the issues surrounding supplements.

In 1994, Congress passed the Dietary Supplement and Health Education Act, which permits over-the-counter sales of herbal and other types of supplements. The law does not require documented evidence of the efficacy and safety of these supplements, and there is no guarantee of their dosage and purity. Even if a study finds potential benefits from a supplement, you cannot be sure that the brand you buy has the same properties as the one that was studied, because of the lack of regulation. Furthermore, very few controlled studies have examined the use of herbal supplements for arthritis. Many people assume that if a substance is herbal, it is automatically safe. This assumption is not true; some herbal remedies have adverse side effects or can interfere with prescription medications. It is vital that you check with a pharmacist or other trained health care provider who has researched herbal supplement use.

Glucosamine and Chondroitin

The most common supplements are various herbal remedies, glucosamine, and chondroitin. The herbal remedies have many possible modes of action, and people use them primarily for pain relief. Some believe that glucosamine and chondroitin possess joint protection properties, because each is a component of cartilage (a connective tissue in the body).

One study suggests that the use of glucosamine sulfate decreases the loss of cartilage in patients with osteoarthritis of the knee, while other studies demonstrate improved function and pain reduction with doses of 1500mg. per day (Reginster et al. 2001; Noack et al. 1994). Arthritis patients usually take nonsteroidal anti-inflammatory drugs (NSAIDs) to help reduce pain and swelling. Several studies have shown that glucosamine has similar pain-reducing properties, without the adverse side effects of NSAIDs (Müller-Faßbender et al. 1994; Qui et al. 1998). The primary side effect of glucosamine is gastrointestinal upset, and not all people

Risky Supplements

Dietary supplements are not tested as rigorously as medicines, and thus may have harmful effects. They are not necessarily labeled properly, and they may interact with medications you take.

Some of these substances have been linked to heart irregularities, increases in blood pressure, seizures, and even death.

Steer clear of these risky substances:

▷ Ephedrine or ephedra (used in weight loss or energy supplements)

▷ Kava (purported to produce relaxation and reduce sleeplessness)

▷ Prohormones or herbal anabolic supplements, such as androstenedione or yohimbine

Even vitamins and minerals can be toxic if taken in excessive quantities. For example:

▷ Vitamins B_6 and B_{12} can cause liver damage.

▷ Vitamin C can cause stomach upset, interfere with copper and iron levels in the body, and may contribute to the formation of kidney stones.

Check with a knowledgeable person who is qualified to give you information about a supplement before you try it, such as a physician, pharmacist, or registered dietitian.

Consumer Lab has a Web site, www.consumerlab.com, which gives information on supplements.

respond to its use. Although less research exists on chondroitin, studies do provide evidence that chondroitin can reduce pain in people using 1200 mg. per day.

Several people tell me how beneficial glucosamine has been for them. One woman who has difficulty taking NSAIDs swears that glucosamine allows her to keep active. A piano teacher says she can tell the difference when she does not take glucosamine. Glucosamine seems to be most effective for those who have mild to moderate arthritis, and it may be worth trying because of the reduced side effects.

Fish Oil

Fish oil is a nutritional supplement that has shown some promising beneficial effects for patients with rheumatoid arthritis. It is high in omega-3 and omega-6 fatty acids, which may have anti-inflammatory effects. In studies, patients who took a supplement of fish oil reported decreased pain. No serious side effects were noted; thus, this supplement may be worth trying if you are looking for alternative pain relief (Tidow-Kebritchi and Mobarhan 2001; Curtis et al. 2002; Calder 2002).

Calcium

Calcium is essential for bone and muscle health and is found in numerous foods. Many people, however, do not get enough calcium in their diets. If these people are at risk for osteoporosis, they may need a calcium supplement. In fact, one text notes that "calcium remains one of the most frequently lacking nutrients in the diet for both non-athlete and athlete" (McArdle, Katch, and Katch 2000, p. 77). Vitamin D, which is often low in older people, facilitates calcium absorption. Therefore, you may require a supplement that contains both calcium and vitamin D.

The recommended dietary allowance for men and women between the ages of 20 and 50 is 1000 milligrams (abbreviated as mg) of calcium and 5 micrograms (abbreviated as mcg) of vitamin D (the requirements are higher during pregnancy and lactation). The calcium requirement increases to 1200 mg after age 50. For vitamin D, the recommendation increases to 10 mcg between 51 and 70 years of age and to 15 mcg after the age of 70 (National Academy of Sciences 2001). These two supplements do not decrease pain, but they should help maintain bone density and proper muscle contractile properties.

Weight Management

Although the focus of this book is on exercise, basic nutrition and weight management affect joint and muscle health, and thus need to be addressed briefly. Obesity is a primary risk factor for developing arthritis, and even moderately overweight people develop knee arthritis more often than those who maintain normal weight (Felson and Zhang 1998). Weight loss can slow joint deterioration and pain. In fact, one study showed that a loss of 11 pounds decreased the risk of developing arthritis symptoms by 50 percent (Felson et al. 1992).

Exercise combined with dietary modification is the best way to lose body fat and improve your health. Radical diets may result in rapid weight loss, but studies have repeatedly proven that such diets are ineffective over the long run. Small, sustainable changes in basic diet are usually healthier, because they do not have a yo-yo effect on weight. Dietary guidelines focus on good, simple steps for a healthy diet (U.S. Department of Health and Human Services 2000). The guidelines include the following:

- Use the food pyramid as a guide to food selection.
- Choose sensible portions.
- Eat a variety of grains, fruits, and vegetables.

- Eat a diet low in saturated fats and cholesterol.
- Moderate your intake of sugars.

The American Dietetic Association has additional suggestions:

- Eat regular meals.
- Reduce, do not eliminate, your intake of certain foods.
- Balance your food choices over time.
- Know your diet pitfalls.

Some of these common sense recommendations are central for preserving health and making dietary changes. Skipping meals decreases concentration and can alter your body's regulation of sugar and food storage. As a result, you may find yourself eating too much when you do sit down to eat, or even storing more fat instead of losing any. One of the problems with some strict diets is that you must give up many foods, including ones that you really like. Many people feel they will not or cannot diet because of such strictures, or if they do try to diet, they eventually give up. The suggestion that you do not give up favorite foods but eat them less often, and in smaller portions, allows you to enjoy your diet instead of resent it.

The food pyramid, developed by the U.S. Department of Agriculture, is shown in figure 7.2. It identifies the nutritional groups and the number

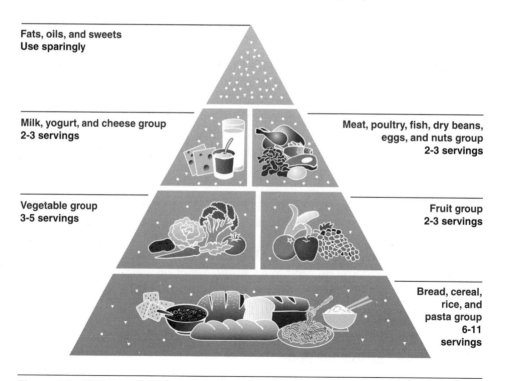

Figure 7.2 USDA Food Guide Pyramid.

Source: U.S. Department of Agriculture/U.S. Department of Health and Human Services.

of servings recommended for each group. An important clarification is what constitutes a serving within each group. Table 7.1 lists sample servings. One way of making sure that you get a variety of foods from different groups is to select a variety of colors for each meal. For example, if you have a meal with baked chicken, mashed potatoes, and baked beans, the color scheme is bland—cream to brown. None of these foods is bad; they simply do not provide enough variety. If you substitute broccoli for the beans, you start to increase the color spectrum and thereby expand the selection from the pyramid.

A common contributor to excessive weight is taking portions that are too large; hence the guideline of choosing sensible portions. Even active athletes can have weight control problems, resulting from difficulty with choosing sensible portions. Exercise is a vital component of any weight management program, and it is most effective when combined with an appropriate diet.

As noted in the previous section, calcium is a valuable nutritional component for someone who is exercising and has arthritis. Good sources of

Table 7.1   Examples of Single-Serving Sizes for Each Food Group

Breads, cereal, rice, and pasta group	Fruit group
1 slice bread	1 piece fruit or melon wedge
1 tortilla	1 cup fruit juice
1/2 cup cooked rice, pasta, or cereal	1/2 cup chopped, cooked, or canned fruit
1 oz. ready-to-eat cereal	1/4 cup dried fruit
1/2 hamburger roll, bagel, or English muffin	**Milk, yogurt, and cheese group**
3-4 plain crackers (small)	1 cup milk or yogurt
1 pancake	1 1/2 oz. natural cheese
Vegetable group	2 oz. process cheese
	1 cup cottage cheese
1/2 cup chopped raw or cooked vegetables	1 cup ice cream or ice milk
1 cup raw leafy vegetables	1 cup frozen yogurt
3/4 cup vegetable juice	**Meat, poultry, fish, dry beans, eggs, and nuts group**
1/2 cup scalloped potatoes	
1/2 cup potato salad	2 1/2 to 3 oz. cooked lean beef, pork, lamb, veal, poultry, or fish
10 french fries	1/2 cup cooked beans = 1 oz. meat
	1 egg = 1 oz. meat
	2 tbsp. peanut butter = 1 oz. meat
	1/3 cup nuts = 1 oz. meat

calcium are milk, yogurt, and cheeses. Some fish (sardines and salmon) and vegetables (such as collards and broccoli) are also good calcium sources.

If you have problems maintaining a well-balanced diet, a registered dietitian can help. They can analyze your diet, identify nutritional deficits or excesses, and make specific recommendations for improving your eating habits. The section on resources at the end of the book lists several nutritional resources to help you find appropriate information and help.

Selecting Your Joint Protection Means

Several ways to protect joints have been suggested, some comprehensive and some joint specific. The question now is which ones are appropriate for you. Some of these methods apply to everyone, and I strongly encourage you to incorporate them into your life. They include proper posture, appropriate shoes, and healthy diet.

Few people have ideal posture, yet it is relatively simple to make it better. Start by doing an overall analysis of your standing and sitting posture. Select one or two aspects to focus on, such as head and shoulder position. Next, identify a few visual or physical cues that you can use to reinforce proper posture. For example, when you walk, looking straight ahead (visual reinforcement) helps to position your head over your trunk. Every time you pass a mirror, check to see if your head and shoulders are up and slightly back. When I am driving, I use the headrest as a physical cue that my head is over my trunk; my head must be touching the headrest for proper alignment. Since posture is a factor in neck and back pain, tackling faulty posture may help decrease symptoms for those of you who suffer this sort of discomfort.

I have repeatedly emphasized the importance of proper shoes for exercise, especially if you have lower-extremity arthritis. Check your shoes at the beginning of each month, and if they are starting to look worn, replace them immediately. Do not wait until they are falling apart, which is likely to happen at the same time that you develop symptoms of pain or injury due to inadequate foot support. One gentleman that I treated had superglued his sole together several times, and his toes had worn holes in the top of the shoe. Shortly after replacing his shoes, his symptoms subsided. Also, as mentioned earlier, do not buy a shoe because it is the cheapest one. Make sure the shoe meets your support needs and is appropriate for the exercise that you are doing.

You may think that diet management is not necessary because your weight is normal. However, I know very few people who have an ideal diet, myself included. Diet management applies to everyone. If your weight is normal and you eat a well-balanced diet, you may simply need to monitor your diet. If you do not have good eating habits or need to lose a bit of weight, then you should spend some time on this area.

Usually the first step when looking at nutrition is to analyze your present diet. In the resource list at the end of the book, I list the Web site for the U.S. Department of Agriculture, which features an interactive program for analyzing your diet. Not only does it analyze your eating habits, you can also keep track of your diet and monitor changes. After analyzing your nutritional intake, identify areas that are weak and one or two changes that address that weakness. This process is similar to baseline testing for fitness and identifying your goals. Make small changes and, just as with exercise, monitor your progress. Again, if you find major deficiencies, you may wish to contact a registered dietitian to get expert help.

Supplements, although global in their effect, are an individual choice. Discuss them with your physician before taking any supplements. Most physicians do not discourage the use of glucosamine, since it appears to cause no serious side effects and since many individuals find that it delivers significant pain relief. If your pain is relieved by taking glucosamine instead of nonsteroidal anti-inflammatories, do so; the side effects are fewer, and the potential for maintaining cartilage health is a bonus.

Specific joint protection devices can cause more damage than they prevent if used incorrectly or not fitted properly. For most of them, you need to consult your physician or other health care specialist. You can try a few over-the-counter devices during the early stages of arthritis, such as flexible wrist supports or heel cushions. Since they have a limited effect on joint mechanics, the potential for damage is also minor. The key to determining whether you need a device is the amount and type of stress you place on the joint. Braces are probably most necessary if you engage in an activity that stresses the joint by rotating or sideways movements, such as tennis or skiing. In any case, neither an over–the-counter device nor a custom-fit apparatus prescribed by your physician should increase your joint pain. If it does, something is wrong and needs to be corrected.

Once you choose exercises and joint protection strategies, you are ready to participate in an exercise program and reap all of the benefits that come with it. In the next chapter, I will discuss some ideas to help you stick with your program once you have gotten started. Even the most dedicated athletes confront potential breaks in their training. The key to success is preventing those training stoppers that you can, and coming back quickly from those that you cannot prevent.

ACTION PLAN:
PROTECTING YOUR JOINTS

☐ Check your posture. Make sure that

- a vertical line could pass through your ear, the tip of your shoulder, the middle of your hip, the back of your knee, and the front of your ankle;
- your spine is in neutral;
- your chest is out;
- your head and shoulders are pulled back over your trunk; and
- your head is up (look straight ahead).

☐ Obtain shoes that are supportive and comfortable.

☐ Determine whether you need splints for problem joints.

☐ Look into supplement use, but get information and consult with your doctor.

☐ Assess your diet and alter it as necessary using the guidelines given.

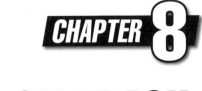

CHAPTER 8

STAYING ON TRACK

Designing a program is not too difficult once you learn some basic principles, and starting the program, although not easy, is often supported by enthusiasm for a new venture. Sticking with a program is where most people have problems. A woman with whom I work restarts her exercise programs at least twice a year. Reasons not to exercise are always popping up—she had surgery on her foot, sprained an ankle, was involved in a car accident, and caught the illness that was going around the office. That she stopped her program is understandable; the important point is that she got started again once she had recovered.

Staying on track does not mean that you exercise regardless of complications; it means stick with your program over the long haul, adapting it to the expected and the unexpected. Sometimes you will not be able to continue your regular exercise routine, especially when you have arthritis. The key is modifying it when you need to and getting back into a routine as soon as possible.

Improving Exercise Adherence

You can use several methods to maintain your adherence to an exercise program. In chapter 1, I suggest that you identify support mechanisms—ways to encourage yourself to stick with your program. Some of these elements must be addressed before you begin a program, such as a facility's location and accessibility, convenient times to work out, and individuals who will either exercise with you or reinforce your participation in a program. Other strategies for continuing to exercise are things you can do once you have started a program. Such strategies anticipate problems and develop alternative exercise routines if, for instance, your arthritis flares up, your partner cannot join you, or some other unplanned change in your routine occurs.

Anticipating Problems

I find that one of the best ways to stay with an exercise program is to anticipate problems ahead of time so that I have a plan for returning to my routine after it has been disrupted. This process can be as simple as expecting that at some point you will miss one or more exercise sessions and identifying a broad plan for returning to activity.

You can also prepare for unexpected setbacks. What will you do if the facility at which you exercise closes, even temporarily? You may not have planned for this specific event, but if you have already worked out an alternate routine, you can fall back on it until you develop a new permanent program. The gym where I do my resistance training is a university facility, so it often closes or alters its hours when the students are on break. I have some small hand and cuff weights, so that I can work out at home whenever necessary. I did not anticipate this exact problem, but I knew there would be days that I could not get into the university and developed a home routine to use at such times.

Think about the past year in relation to your schedule, your health, and any unforeseen occurrences. Using the last year as a guideline, you can anticipate potential breaks in your schedule and develop a plan to deal with them. For example, most people had colds or other temporary illness within the last year. When you do not have fever or a chest infection, physicians often suggest that you continue mild activity, because it helps the immune system. A short walk and flexibility activities are still possible; you can even walk indoors. With a more severe illness, you need rest and should stop most of your exercise routine. Range of motion activities are still feasible, and they help fend off the increased stiffness that often accompanies bed rest.

Dealing With a Flare-up

For a person with arthritis, one of the most common problems that interferes with exercise is an arthritic flare-up. The stiffness, joint pain, and inflammation that are the hallmarks of arthritis can vary from day to day. When one or more of these symptoms increases significantly and quickly, you need to adapt your program. Furthermore, during flare-ups your immune system is compromised; if you put additional stress on the system by exercising, your symptoms may become worse or you may become ill.

The first and simplest adaptation is to decrease the intensity and frequency of your exercise regimen. Resistance training puts the greatest amount of stress on joints, so cut back on your strength-training routine. You should also reduce the intensity of your cardiovascular program; I suggest that you use perceived exertion as a way of determining how hard to work and that you exercise in the mild range.

While lowering the intensity of your exercise program, you also need to increase your rest. Earlier I discussed the importance of both general and joint-specific rest. Extended rest during a flare-up allows your body to direct extra energy toward healing, and you will feel better sooner. Eliminating joint-specific activity that increases your pain allows that joint to recover. Remember, the amount of rest you need depends on the severity of your illness. Usually you can continue to do some activity (at reduced intensity), since low-intensity activity helps the immune system and wards off excessive joint stiffness. Complete rest of either type should not last long, or you will lose mobility and strength very quickly.

In addition to modifying your exercise plan, consider using extra protection for your joints. During flare-ups, joints may be unstable, because the tissues surrounding the joints become inflamed. If you cannot modify an

Activity-Related Injury Care

Not all activity-related injuries can be prevented. If you do injure yourself, the following very general guidelines can help you. If you cannot put weight or pressure on the injured limb (such as standing on a leg), if the pain is extreme or does not subside, or there is a noticeable deformity, you should see a physician.

For acute injuries such as ankle sprains or pulled muscles apply the "RICE" prescription:

R = Rest: Stop intense activity until the pain decreases; use gentle range of motion to keep the area from stiffening.

I = Ice: Ice the area for up to 20 minutes every 2 to 3 hours for the first 48 hours following the injury.

C = Compression: Wrap the ankle or area with a gentle compression wrap to decrease swelling, usually for the first 48 hours.

E = Elevation: If possible, rest with the limb elevated, which will help to decrease swelling.

After 48 hours, depending on the severity of injury, you can start putting more weight on the limb and slowly increase the intensity of your activity. Heat may help with residual stiffness and will improve circulation to the area.

Overuse injuries develop over time and include problems such as tendinitis and bursitis. Treatment includes rest, decreased activity, or an alternative activity. Heat may help with stiffness and circulation. Before returning to the activity, check your shoes and biomechanics, as these often contribute to overuse.

Following any injury it is important to strengthen the muscles around the injury and to make sure that range of motion is normal.

activity to decrease stress on the joint, it's a good idea to splint or brace the joint to protect it from further injury. Chapter 7 discusses ideas for joint protection, ranging from simple devices (such as neoprene sleeves) to complex braces. If you are going to be putting a significant amount of stress on an involved joint, you should discuss options with your physician. A man I know insisted on continuing the downhill skiing season, even though his knee had become extremely swollen, painful, and unstable. Although the ideal solution would have been to give up skiing for the season, he was willing to wear a brace, which gave some protection and reminded him of his joint limitations. At the end of the season he had joint replacement surgery, so that his next ski season would not be affected.

Finally, you can use several modalities to decrease the swelling and pain associated with arthritis. Usually your physician will advise you to take an anti-inflammatory, especially during flare-ups. The use of cold or heat will alleviate some of the pain. In general, use cold when there is noticeable swelling, but it does increase tissue stiffness. Heat may increase inflammation, but it also increases tissue flexibility. Talk to your physician before you use either heat or cold; you should not use them if you have certain circulatory problems.

Flexible Programming

When you thought back over the last year, there were the unanticipated breaks in activity, such as already discussed, and you probably had some changes that could have been anticipated. Instead of waiting for that bad weather day and skipping your routine because it isn't feasible, plan ahead. Come up with some alternative workout regimens that you can slip into your routine when necessary. Note that I didn't wait for the gym where I workout to alter its hours, I had a backup routine that I could do at home. The two most common breaks to routine that you can anticipate are trips and bad weather.

Traveling

I am sometimes asked, "How can I exercise when I am away from home?" You have several alternatives, depending on where you are going and what facilities are available at your destination. Investigate your destination beforehand. If you are staying at a hotel or resort, they can often give you the information you need ahead of time. Ask the following questions:

1. Are exercise facilities available on-site? If so, does it cost extra to use them? What do the facilities include?
2. Is it safe to walk or run outside in the area?
3. Are there any trails or routes nearby, and how long are they?
4. Are there any facilities nearby that offer short-term access?

Some of these questions may sound nit-picky, but I have learned through experience that even with specific inquiries, the answers and the reality may not be the same. I have been in hotels where I was told they had a well-equipped exercise room, only to find one treadmill, a bike, and an exercise mat. Another resort advertised "extensive walking trails on the grounds"; it turned out that they were counting the cart paths for the golf course—not a very safe place to walk during the golf season.

Once you have answered these questions, develop a tentative workout schedule. Without a schedule, it is very easy to put your exercise session off until the next day (if you do it at all). The easiest cardiovascular exercises to do while traveling are usually walking and running, so you need to know about the safety of the area and available routes. When traveling to new towns walking or running can be a nice way to discover the lay of the land. If you do not have a map that indicates mileage, or measured routes, then use duration to guide your workout.

If the area is not safe for outdoor exercise, you can do an indoor regimen. Facilities that are in-house or nearby may provide safe alternatives. Sometimes local facilities allow visitors temporary access; they may even offer short-term memberships. When you end up staying in an area that is not considered safe, and no other facilities are available, you can do a modified routine in your room, marching or jogging in place for a short period.

Plan a modified strength program that uses body weight activities or rubber tubing. Good basic body weight moves include abdominal crunches, push-ups, birddog exercises, and wall sits. These four exercises work your arms, shoulders, trunk, and lower extremities, and they can be done every day. Rubber tubing is great for traveling, since it is light and portable. You can perform a simple resistance program every other day. Biceps and triceps curls combined with extension and flexion exercises for the hip and knee make up a good routine that does not take long. You may not have tubing thick enough to provide a high resistance, so focus on muscular endurance and do more repetitions.

Stiffness can become more troublesome when you travel, because you do a good deal more sitting than usual. Therefore, do not sacrifice your flexibility routine, even if you occasionally have to miss the other two components of your program. Most people with whom I work find it easiest to divide their flexibility programs into two parts—range of motion exercises in the morning to loosen up, and both range of motion and stretching activities in the evening, before retiring. In addition, work in some range of motion movements whenever you have been sitting for a prolonged period. I go to a sports medicine conference every year, during which I go from meeting to meeting, often sitting for most of the day. In between each session I do some shoulder rolls, reach for the sky moves, and even short stretches for my hamstrings and calves. If you will be driving or sitting in a car for a long time, try to plan regular rest stops during which you can do some stretching and moving.

You must make two key preparations to maintain a program when you are traveling. The first is making some alternative exercise plans. The second is being flexible with your plans. You may have the best intentions to keep up your exercise routine, but your travel schedule does not always allow you to stick to your plans. Remember, even a 10-minute walk is better than nothing, and if you miss a day, you can get back on track the next day.

Inclement Weather

Bad weather can present a barrier to exercise in more than one way. On some days you cannot safely do outdoor exercise (such as during severe thunderstorms), or it simply is not appealing. I live in a snowbelt in the Midwest; on several days during the winter, it is either too icy or too cold to exercise safely outside. In fact, I can count on there being one or two days when I cannot even drive to a facility. A backup plan for such days is key to maintaining your program. Choose an alternate place to exercise or another type of exercise. Several years ago I asked for an indoor cross-country ski machine, which I use during the winter when I cannot get outdoors. Some of you may suffer greater stiffness in the cold and so may use an indoor program throughout the winter. A patient with whom I once worked found that with a note from her physician, she could gain access to a local indoor walking track. She uses this track during inclement or frigid weather and walks outside the rest of the time.

Your backup exercise plan does not have to be elaborate. You can get a good workout using your own body weight, supplemented by either rubber tubing or a few handheld weights. I have rubber tubing, one set of dumbbells, and one set of cuff weights at home. With this equipment, I can do a program that at least helps me to maintain my strength until I can get back to the gym. As with a travel program, you can do basic abdominal crunches, push-ups, and wall sits, which use only your body weight. Using the tubing or small weights, add biceps and triceps curls for your upper body and knee and hip extension and flexion for your lower body. Again, you will probably find it easier to do an endurance type of resistance program—high repetitions and low resistance—with the tubing or small weights. You do not usually need to modify your flexibility program, since these activities are normally done indoors.

Exercising in the Cold

If you plan to exercise outside, prepare for exercising in both the cold and the heat. The primary health risks associated with exercising in the cold are hypothermia and tissue damage. Guard against them by wearing proper clothing that holds in body temperature and does not leave skin exposed. The ACSM has developed guidelines for distance running in extreme temperatures that may help you, even if you are not a runner (ACSM, *Heat and cold,* 1998). Common recommendations regarding exercise in the cold include the following:

1. Dress in layers—the layer closest to the skin should be a material that wicks away moisture from the skin.
2. Wear a head covering to reduce heat loss.
3. Wear a face mask or ski mask to protect the face if temperatures are extremely cold.
4. Cover your nose and mouth with a face mask or scarf if your respiratory system is sensitive to cold.
5. Wear feet and hand coverings made of material that wicks away moisture, and over that wear a layer of water-resistant or waterproof materials (shoes and gloves).
6. Wear mittens rather than gloves to provide more protection against the cold—mittens keep the fingers together, reducing heat loss.

One topic not addressed in the recommendations is how arthritis responds to exercise in the cold. The most common symptom that arthritis manifests during exposure to cold is an increase in stiffness. Exercising, which produces body heat, should reduce this symptom. Further insulation of the joint or area also eases stiffness. You can wear a neoprene sleeve around the joint, as noted earlier, or wear an extra layer of clothing. If you become stiffer with cold weather, increase your warm-up time; you may also need to decrease the intensity of the exercise. Hands and feet can be especially sensitive to the cold. Sporting goods stores, as well as other retailers, sell silk liners. Wearing such liners under wool socks or gloves is both comfortable and warm. Although not necessary for exercise, a variety of devices for warming the hands (often disposable) are available if you are going to be out in the cold and not moving around a great deal.

Exercising in the Heat

Exercising in the heat does not pose the same physiological challenge as exercising in the cold. A vital concern during exercise is heat loss, which decreases with high temperatures and humidity. If your body is unable to lose heat, body core temperature starts to rise and you are at risk for heat illness, which can be life-threatening. Guidelines for exercise in the heat are the following:

1. Avoid strenuous exercise when the temperature is high (above 90 degrees Fahrenheit), especially if the relative humidity is also high (greater than 60 percent).
2. Wear light, absorbent clothing.

3. Cover your head to decrease absorption of radiant heat.

4. Exercise early in the morning or late in the evening, when the radiant temperature is not as high.

5. Decrease intensity of exercise and monitor yourself for signs and symptoms of heat-related problems.

(ACSM, *Heat and cold,* 1998; Hoeger and Hoeger 2002)

Arthritis problems related to exercising in the heat are different than those encountered in the cold. They are more likely to occur if you have a systemic type of arthritis, such as rheumatoid arthritis, or other systemic disease. In such cases your heat loss mechanisms may not function as well, meaning you may be more susceptible to heat-related illness. It is true that heat may reduce stiffness, but other systems (such as your cardiovascular system) may not adjust as well. Following sensible guidelines becomes even more important, and you should consider alternative exercise routines.

Joint Replacement Surgery

As arthritis progresses, your affected joints lose motion, even with regular exercise, and may eventually become deformed. Fortunately, modern joint replacement techniques are now available when joint integrity breaks down and pain becomes severe. At some point, your physician may suggest joint replacement surgery for you. Nobody likes the idea of surgery, but putting off the surgery too long can prolong your rehabilitation. I have had many patients in the hospital who were not able to go home after joint replacement surgery; they had to go instead to an interim care facility, because they were too weak on the nonsurgical side to move themselves in and out of a chair or bed. You can speed up your recovery by doing a presurgery exercise program. I will focus here on lower-extremity joint surgery, because this type of surgery affects mobility the most.

Presurgery Preparation

Before my aunt's hip operation and my father's knee surgery, I told each that they needed to prepare their bodies for rehabilitation. Both of them told me later that doing the exercises I suggested before going into the hospital had proven very helpful. Two essential goals for people facing surgery are maintaining cardiovascular fitness and building strength. Cardiovascular fitness improves your overall recovery, while strength enables you to perform functions that you might currently take for granted. If your joint has become so aggravated that you have difficulty doing your normal aerobic activity, you need to identify an alternative, at least until the surgery. Keep doing some walking, since this is a functional activity and one that you will be doing after surgery.

I emphasize simple strength exercises that focus on two functions: the ability to rise from sitting to standing position using primarily one leg, and the ability to support your body weight (with arm strength) while using a walker or crutches. You will be in better shape for surgery if you are already doing some strengthening activities as part of your fitness program. If not, these exercises are even more crucial. For lower-extremity strength, I suggest a combination of wall sits, straight leg raises, and sit-to-stand practice using a single leg.

One of the modifications I suggested to my dad was the single leg wall slide—a partial squat with the back against the wall, using one leg. It is more difficult than a regular wall sit, but it is an excellent strengthener, which you can do in sets of 10 repetitions. Concentrate on strengthening the leg that will not be having surgery, but if possible, also do the exercise with the leg that will undergo surgery. For any of the single-leg exercises, hold on to a stable chair or other heavy object.

The straight leg raise is actually designed for neural activation, so you can perform sets of 15 repetitions. You must be able to perform this motion after surgery in order to get your leg off the bed for transferring and other activities. To progress this exercise, add a small cuff weight to your ankle, as long as it does not irritate your knee. You can do these strength activities at home every day before your surgery.

If you have rubber tubing, add some strength exercises for your hamstrings, quadriceps, and hips, using the more traditional strengthening guidelines discussed in chapter 4. I recommend that you do knee extension and flexion movements—either the closed chain standing exercise or the open chain sitting exercise will work. To strengthen the hips so that they can support you during transfers and walking, do hip extension, flexion, and abduction exercises.

Single-Leg Wall Squat

Stand with your back against the wall and your legs about 2 feet away from it, shoulder width apart. Hold on to the back of a chair or other stable object for support, and raise one foot off the ground. While keeping that foot raised, slowly lower your trunk toward a sitting position, using the wall for support (see figure 8.1). Hold the end position for a few seconds, then slide back to standing. Repeat this movement 10 times.

Straight Leg Raise

Lie on your back on the floor (or on your bed, if you cannot manage the floor easily). Bend one leg and place that foot flat on the floor. Lift the other leg, keeping your knee straight, to about 45 degrees (see figure 8.2). Then slowly lower your leg back to the floor or bed. Perform this movement with both legs.

You also need upper-extremity strength when facing surgery. After surgery you will be walking with a walker or crutches, depending on

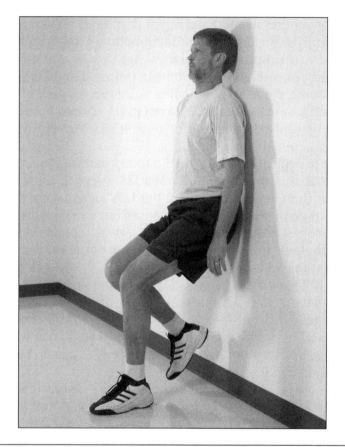

Figure 8.1 Single-leg wall squat.

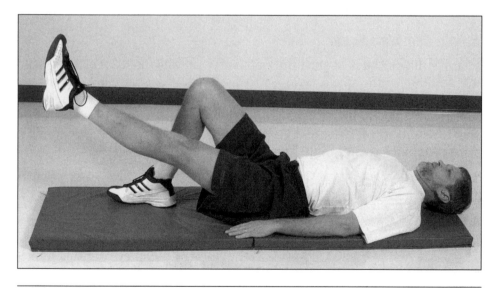

Figure 8.2 Straight leg raise.

your strength and balance and on your physician's instructions. The object in using these assistive devices is to eliminate or decrease the amount of weight placed on your surgical leg. Your arms, aided by the walker or crutches, help support your body weight while you move that leg forward. An easy exercise, which simulates the motion your arms will be doing, is a seated press-up. Start with sets of 5 repetitions, gradually increasing to 10, and repeat the movement two to three times during the day. More traditional upper-body strength exercises include biceps and triceps curls with free weights or tubing and latissimus pull-downs (the latissimus muscles help hold your arms into your sides, a critical skill for walking with crutches).

Seated Press-Up

Sit on a firm, stable chair with your hands curled in a partial fist, so that the tops of your fists are on the chair (beside your hips) and your wrists are straight. Completely straighten your arms, so that your bottom lifts off the chair. You can modify this exercise by using the arm rests to push on (see figure 8.3).

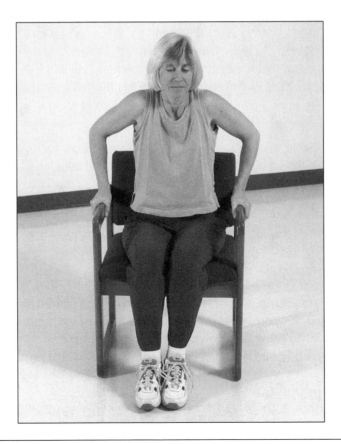

Figure 8.3 Seated press-up.

If possible, it is wise to take care of equipment needs and possible home modifications before you go into the hospital, so that you have one less problem to deal with when you prepare to return home. I have addressed some of these concerns, which include your assistive aid (walker or crutches), rugs, chairs, and bathroom modifications, at the end of the next section, and I have highlighted a few key concerns in the sidebar.

Setting Up Your Home Before Surgery

Many times people do not consider making changes in the home environment until after surgery. If you can address some of these issues beforehand, your return home will be easier.

▷ Who will be available to help you at home, especially during the first week after surgery? Although you may be quite independent, having someone help with chores, meals, and even exercises makes your recovery much easier.

▷ Remove throw rugs and other obstacles on the floor, as a safety precaution.

▷ Will you need assistive aids? If you can get these before the surgery, they can be ready to use when you get home. These aids might include a walker, a raised toilet seat, cushions for chairs, a tote bag that fits on the front of the walker, and even something as simple as a lap table.

▷ Does any of the furniture need to be rearranged? Make sure that you have a clear walking path throughout the house.

▷ When possible, it is best to remain on the ground floor for all activities. If you do not have a bed there, do you have a foldout couch?

▷ If your bathroom and shower do not have stable objects such as a cabinet that you can lean on during transfers, consider having grab bars installed.

Post-Surgery

Rehabilitation usually begins the day after surgery, although if your surgery is early in the morning, the staff may want you to try getting into a chair later that day. Everyone responds differently to anesthesia and surgery, but if you have no complications, it is best to get up and moving as soon as possible, even though you may not feel like it. Getting up significantly decreases the risk of blood clots (which is a normal post-surgical risk) and helps your bodily systems return to normal.

Please do not try to get up on your own or with a spouse's aid, unless your spouse knows how to transfer patients. Your therapist will tell you how much weight you can put on your surgical leg and will supervise your rehabilitation program while you are in the hospital. During this time you will usually walk with a walker (several times per day) and do exercises for your surgical leg.

The most common knee exercises include quadriceps sets, straight leg raises, short-arc knee extensions, and range of motion exercises. Following hip replacement, exercise is often focused on hip extension and abduction. The purpose of this program is to get the muscles firing again, since pain inhibits muscle contraction, and to start regaining range of motion. You may think that these goals sound quite easy—you can lift your leg off the ground now, and surely you can do so after the surgery. My father was quite surprised the first day after surgery, when he tried to do his exercises. What had been exceedingly easy two days before was not possible, and he needed help to get his leg off the bed. This weakness is typical, because the nervous system protects the injured site. With repetition of the intended action, normal function slowly returns.

Before going home, make sure you know what exercises to do at home, how much weight you can put on your surgical leg, and what activities you must not yet attempt. The home exercise program is usually similar to the regimen you started while in the hospital, but now you are responsible. I suggest setting a schedule, which will help you adhere to the program. A simple way to keep track of your regimen is to use a calendar and draw three boxes (representing three exercise sessions) on each day. As you complete each session, you can check that box and thus reinforce your regular schedule.

I also recommend doing a few exercises while standing with your walker or leaning against the kitchen counter. Such exercises include hip extension and abduction for both legs. The leg muscles can become tight when you are sitting a lot during your recovery period. Since the hip muscles are central to walking, you need to maintain their range and, if possible, their strength.

Many programs focus on knee flexion, but it is also essential to get knee extension back to normal range. The quadriceps set exercise works on knee extension, and a small rolled-up towel placed under your knee can give you tactile feedback when you are pushing the back of your knee into it properly. You can also use gravity to help develop knee extension. While you are sitting, place you heel on a low stool or coffee table, with nothing under your knee. Try this position for a few minutes at a time. It is not comfortable, and I find that most people feel better when they do some repeated knee flexion afterward to loosen up the knee. In fact, your surgical knee stiffens rather quickly, so do a few extension and flexion movements periodically, or get up and walk every hour or so.

When the hospital discharges you to go home, they should give you a referral for physical therapy. Therapy can take place either at home or in an outpatient facility, depending on where you live and what your insurance covers. If your doctor has mentioned therapy, make sure to ask about it before your discharge.

Getting Ready to Return Home

Go over several questions with your physician, nurse, and therapist before returning home. These questions include, but are not limited to, the following:

▷ What medications will I take, and for how long? What side effects should I be aware of? A blood thinner is commonly prescribed after surgery to reduce the chance of clots, but they also increase bleeding. You need to be careful of bumps, and you may be restricted to using an electric shaver.

▷ What are my activity restrictions, and when do these restrictions end? Restrictions may include lifting, driving, and weight-bearing exercise, among others.

▷ When do I start therapy, and will I do it at home or as an outpatient? Your therapist should give you a home exercise program, similar to the one I have outlined, to do as an adjunct to regular therapy.

▷ What assistive devices do I need and for how long?

▷ How do I take care of the surgical site? Most hospitals will give you handouts about care of the site and any signs or symptoms that you should report to the physician.

One aspect of fitness that people often neglect during the initial recovery period is cardiovascular fitness. Start with short walks, using your assistive device, usually in the house. Most people focus on functional activity—they walk from one room to another to get something. Try to increase the duration either by walking in place for five minutes, if you can put weight on your leg, or by walking the length of the house several times.

Until you can start walking for longer periods, be creative about doing some aerobic activity. If your doctor allows it, you can use a stationary bike (the seat will need to be adjusted for your surgical knee). If you do not have a stationary bike, you can use your arms to get some aerobic exercise. Holding your arms just below shoulder level, pretend you are pedaling with them. As you have probably not used your arms for aerobic exercise before, you will find that you cannot keep it up for long. If you do it several times a day, however, you will gain some aerobic benefits and can probably work up to five minutes per session. As with any exercise, this movement should not cause pain in your shoulders. Once you start walking more easily, gradually increase the time or distance that you walk.

Equipment and Home Modifications

Several simple equipment and home modifications can help you. If you have hip surgery, therapists usually discuss some of these adjustments with you; they are often helpful for knee surgery patients as well. First, arrange to obtain a walker or crutches before you go into the hospital. Most therapists recommend a folding walker if possible, because they are easier to get into vehicles and set aside in small areas. Another option is a rolling walker. This walker has wheels on the front, with a locking device so it will not roll when you are pressing down. Whether you can use one of these depends on how much weight the physician will allow you to put on the surgical site. Make sure that the walker is the proper height for you. The easiest way to check the height is to stand in the walker with your arms hanging at your sides. Your wrists should be at the grip level, so that when your hands are holding the grips, your elbows will be slightly bent. Your therapist will check the fit of your equipment when you are in the hospital and will teach you the proper sequence of movements when using the walker or crutches.

In addition to adjusting the height of the walker, you may want to alter the grip. Sometimes the pressure put through your hands is uncomfortable. Obtain some pipe insulation from the local hardware store and cut it to a length of six to eight inches. Wrap the insulation around each handle, and secure it with duct tape. Crutch grips are usually well padded and do not need this alteration, although some people like to wrap a wash cloth around the grip, again securing it firmly. You might also acquire a carrying device that you can attach to the front of the walker. These accessories are usually small baskets or tote bags. They can be very helpful when you want to bring a few items from one room to another, since you will not have your hands free to carry them.

Finally, consider a few simple home modifications to augment safety and to assist with transfers. If you have hip surgery, your therapist will talk to you about installing a raised toilet seat. It is also a good idea to raise the seats in other chairs, which you can easily accomplish by adding firm extra seat cushions to the chairs.

Such modifications are helpful even if you have knee surgery. As I mentioned before, my father is tall (6 feet, 4 inches), so when the family was preparing for his return home after knee surgery, I carried out some of these modifications. We found extra cushions especially useful on the sofa and dining room chairs. Chairs with arms are usually easier to get in and out of, since you can lean on the arms. Otherwise, you may want to rearrange some of the furniture so that you have a stable object to hold on to during transfers. Make sure to remove any loose throw rugs, especially if they are on a tile floor and do not have a nonskid backing.

Bringing It All Together

I have examined some of the common ways people get off track and how to plan ahead for disruptions to one's exercise routine. Once again, be flexible in your planning. If you have to interrupt your program for some reason, cut out only what you have to, and make a plan for resuming the program.

One deterrent to exercise that I have not addressed is more difficult to pin down—the "I just don't feel like it today" problem. Again, you need to be flexible and decide whether it is a one-time difficulty (in which case, a day off might be good for you). If you are fighting that feeling more and more often, then you must decide whether it is fatigue, boredom with your program, or some other stressor that might be influencing you. A subtle increase in your arthritis may be draining you before you are aware of it. Try increasing your rest a bit and decreasing the intensity of your workouts. You can alter your program to make it more interesting, and (as mentioned in other chapters) exercising with someone else can give you a big boost. Work and other potential stressors are sometimes the culprit, in which case you will usually feel better if you force yourself to exercise.

A word of caution is in order—do not ignore an increase in fatigue. Even if you can identify a potential cause for your fatigue, such as stress, the problem is no less important. In chapter 1, I discussed the importance of rest, both general and joint-specific. Fatigue can be a sign of a depleted immune system that is unable to provide full resistance against arthritis-related problems. If you have addressed potential causes of fatigue and do not feel better with increased rest, call your physician. Unusual fatigue is a sign that something is wrong.

Staying on track with exercise is never easy, and arthritis adds another potential barrier. I have suggested several ideas to make sticking with your exercise program easier. Keys to staying on track with exercise include the following:

1. Set realistic goals and objectives, and review them on a regular basis.
2. Keep an exercise log to track progress toward your goals.
3. Develop a support system—either exercise partners or reinforcers.
4. Develop a simple, balanced routine that you really like.
5. Be flexible in your approach to an exercise program—adapt elements as your arthritis symptoms require.
6. Be your own expert on arthritis and exercise. Identify reliable resources and learn as much as you can, so that you are in control.

Above all else, I hope that this book helps you realize that arthritis is not a reason to give up exercise. In fact, exercise is one of the best prescriptions for arthritis, helping to decrease pain, increase mobility, and improve self-esteem. I hope that you have found some useful tips for altering your current program or designing a new one.

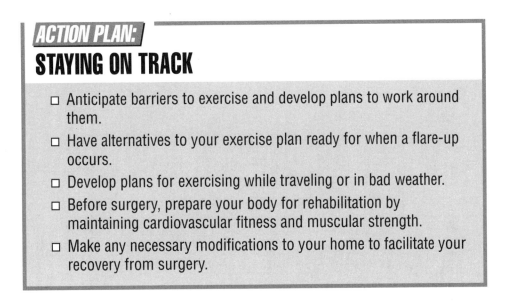

ACTION PLAN:

STAYING ON TRACK

- ☐ Anticipate barriers to exercise and develop plans to work around them.
- ☐ Have alternatives to your exercise plan ready for when a flare-up occurs.
- ☐ Develop plans for exercising while traveling or in bad weather.
- ☐ Before surgery, prepare your body for rehabilitation by maintaining cardiovascular fitness and muscular strength.
- ☐ Make any necessary modifications to your home to facilitate your recovery from surgery.

RESOURCES

Numerous resources on arthritis are available at local, state, and national levels. The state and national resources may have programs offered at local levels. They usually have information on arthritis-related issues that is available through publications and brochures as well as over the Internet. I have listed some of the best-known national resources at the end of this section.

Local Resources

Local hospitals and health groups often offer educational seminars and classes on arthritis and exercise. They may also sponsor support groups for people with arthritis. Usually the people running these programs are trained health care professionals and thus are well qualified. Over the past year, I have seen advertisements almost every month for seminars on arthritis-related topics at local facilities. Topics range from pain management to alternative medicine.

Another potential resource is your local newspaper. Most papers have a health and fitness section; my local newspaper publishes one weekly. Not only do they feature articles devoted to health and exercise, but they often have contact names and numbers for people who write on health-related issues. Such writers often welcome suggestions for topics to research and write about, if you are looking for information on a particular subject. The lead story in a recent health section in my newspaper was devoted to fibromyalgia; it featured a local woman and her battle with this form of arthritis. The article identified potential treatments, along with the regimen that she had found most beneficial, which included stretching and tai chi. The story identified the local fibromyalgia support group and where it met. Libraries are also excellent reference sources, carrying books (usually in the 600s classification of the non-fiction section), magazines, and videos related to health and fitness.

Finally, your local YMCA and other fitness facilities may run exercise classes for individuals with arthritis. As noted in chapter 7, the YMCA offers nationally standardized aerobics classes (both in and out of the pool). Even if there is not a YMCA in your area, other sorts of places may have excellent classes. A facility where I live, designed for people with developmental disabilities, has a warm pool and offers water aerobics for people with arthritis. Other opportunities may be available; my local university has an indoor track that is open at different times throughout the day for older people or people with medical concerns. Because it is a larger facility, stationary bikes and treadmills are also available for exercise.

My list identifies organizations that provide quality, unbiased information that is accessible to everyone. The arthritis-related groups often produce brochures on numerous topics related to arthritis, and some have developed exercise programs that are available at locations throughout the country. Several of the other organizations listed produce information on specialized topics, such as nutrition or exercise. I have also identified the types of information that each group distributes.

One of the concerns I have as a professor and a health care professional is the reliability of the many sorts of materials you may come across. A few years ago, a health care group examined the information presented on various Internet sites about one specific topic. It found that approximately 40 percent of the information was inaccurate. So, how can you decide whether a source of information is credible? Whether it is an Internet article, a book, or a video, asking the following questions can help you evaluate a resource:

1. Is the resource associated with or endorsed by a reputable national organization? Examples include government-sponsored Web sites, or materials from well-respected organizations such as the YMCA.

2. Does the article or text list references that provide evidence for statements they make, or are they able to give such references on request? A reputable source either cites references or is willing to provide them.

3. Are the references from a variety of sources? When the references all refer to obscure journals or "unpublished data," it is a red flag.

4. Does the author seem to be promoting himself and his approach as the only one? Having read this book, you can appreciate that many different approaches to exercising with arthritis are successful.

Foundations and Informational Groups

Arthritis Foundation
P.O. Box 7669
Atlanta, GA 30357-0669
Phone: 800-283-7800
www.arthritis.org
> Brochures: Exercise and Arthritis (series)
> Courses: Arthritis Self-Help Course

Arthritis Society
393 University Ave., Ste. 1700
Toronto, ON M5G 1E6
Phone: 800-321-1433
www.arthritis.ca
Brochures

National Institute of Arthritis and Musculoskeletal and Skin Diseases
1 AMS Circle
Bethesda, MD 20892
877-22-NIAMS
www.nih.gov/niams
Publications on exercise and arthritis

American College of Rheumatology
1800 Century Plaza, Ste. 250
Atlanta, GA 30345-4300
Phone: 404-633-3777
www.rheumatology.org
Publications on exercise

Missouri Arthritis Rehabilitation Research & Training Center
130 A P Green, DC330.00
One Hospital Drive
Columbia, MO 65212
www.muhealth.org/~arthritis
Video: Good Moves for Everybody
Publications on exercise

National Osteoporosis Foundation
1150 17th St. NW, Ste. 500
Washington, DC 20036
Phone: 202-223-2226
www.nof.org
Brochures on exercise

Centers for Disease Control and Prevention
1600 Clifton Rd.
Atlanta, GA 30333
Phone: 800-311-3435
www.cdc.gov
Publications on arthritis and exercise

National Institute on Aging Information Center
Bldg. 31, Rm. 5C27
Bethesda, MD 20892
Phone: 800-222-2225
www.nih.gov/nia
Publications

Department of Health and Human Services
Administration on Aging
Washington, DC 20201
Phone: 202-619-0724
www.aoa.gov
Brochures

American Dietetic Association
120 S. Riverside Plaza, Ste. 2000
Chicago, IL 60606-6995
Phone: 312-899-0040
www.eatright.org
Brochures
Nutrition hot line

National Center for Nutrition and Dietetics
216 W. Jackson Blvd.
Chicago, IL 60606-6995
Nutrition hot line: 800-366-1655

U.S. Department of Agriculture
Center for Nutrition Policy and Promotion
www.usda.gov/cnpp
Interactive Healthy Eating Index
www.health.gov/dietaryguidelines

International Food Information Council Foundation
1100 Connecticut Ave. NW, Ste. 430
Washington, DC 20036
www.ificinfo.health.org
Numerous brochures

American Academy of Orthopedic Surgeons
P.O. Box 1998
Des Plaines, IL 60017
Phone: 800-346-2267
www.aaos.org
   Publications on exercise, joint replacement

American College of Sports Medicine
401 W. Michigan St.
Indianapolis, IN 46202-3233
Phone: 317-637-9200
www.acsm.org
   Brochures: Selecting a stationary cycle, selecting a treadmill

American Physical Therapy Association
111 N. Fairfax St.
Alexandria, VA 22314-1488
Phone: 800-999-2782
www.apta.org
   Brochures on exercise

National Council for Reliable Health Information (NCRHI)
P.O. Box 1276
Loma Linda, CA 92354
www.ncahf.org
   Information on reliability of health claims, Web sites

GLOSSARY

abduction—Movement away from the midline of the body, for example, lifting the arm out to the side.

adduction—Movement toward, or across, the midline of the body, such as bringing one leg toward the other leg.

aerobic—Requiring oxygen; usually refers to exercise that needs oxygen at the cellular level to produce energy.

anaerobic—Oxygen not required; usually refers to the ability of the muscle cells to produce energy without oxygen.

articular cartilage—A special type of tissue that covers the ends of bones and allows smooth movement between the bones in a joint. It also absorbs force during movement.

biceps—Muscle on the front of the upper arm; it bends the elbow and helps flex the shoulder.

biomechanics—The application of mechanical principles to the study of human movement.

cardiovascular endurance—The ability of the heart to deliver oxygen to the working muscles, and the muscles' ability to use that oxygen.

circuit training—Performance of exercises in an alternating sequence; used mostly with resistance exercises, though aerobic exercises can be put within the sequence.

closed chain—Movement of a limb during which the hand or foot is kept in contact with either the ground or a device that has a prescribed motion, such as a bicycle pedal. Because of the "fixed" extremity, the movements of each joint within that limb are predictable.

concentric—A muscle contraction during which the joint angle becomes smaller and the muscle appears to shorten.

deltoid—Muscle that goes from the top of the arm to the trunk. There are three parts to this muscle, which is involved in raising the arm and in extending and flexing the shoulder.

eccentric—A muscle contraction during which the joint angle becomes greater and the muscle appears to lengthen.

extension—Movement which straightens a joint, for example, the knee when coming from sit to stand. Extension for the shoulder and hip refer to motion which moves the limb behind the body, such as reaching backward.

fartlek training—A Swedish term meaning "speed play"; the aerobic training session is continuous with varied speeds throughout.

flare-up—A temporary increase in stiffness and joint pain associated with arthritis; may include swelling as well.

flexibility—Refers to the ability of a joint (or joints) to move throughout its complete range, which is dictated by the muscles that cross that joint.

flexion—Movement which bends a joint, such as the elbow when the arm is bent.

functional fitness—The ability to perform normal daily activities around the house or at work, without undue fatigue.

hamstrings—Group of three muscles on the back of the thigh. These muscles bend the knee and help to extend the hip.

hyperthermia—High body temperature; life-threatening if uncontrolled.

hypothermia—Low body temperature; life-threatening if uncontrolled.

impact—The amount of force transmitted through the body upon landing.

inflammation—Swelling that occurs within joints, muscles, or spaces within tissues.

interval training—A form of training that uses alternating periods of rest or lower-intensity exercise, and exercise. For example, running a mile, then walking or resting for a predetermined period, then running another mile, and so on.

isometric—A muscle contraction during which no joint movement occurs, for example, when an individual pushes against a wall.

isotonic—A muscle contraction that involves movement of the joint and apparent shortening or lengthening of the muscle.

latissimus dorsi—Large muscle on the back which attaches to the upper arm and is used to pull the arm to the side.

metabolism—The breakdown of food sources to produce energy at the cellular level.

neuromuscular—Refers to the control of muscular activity by the nervous system.

nonsteroidal anti-inflammatory drugs (NSAIDs)—Drugs that are not steroids used to control or decrease swelling. Common examples include over-the-counter drugs such as aspirin and ibuprofen, and prescription drugs such as naproxen and Voltaren.

open chain—Movement during which the hand or foot can move in any direction desired, thus the movement of the joints within that limb are not predictable. An example would be movement of the leg when it is off of the ground.

orthotics—Devices that help control movement at a joint, thus helping to maintain proper mechanical alignment and protect the joint.

oxygen consumption—The use of oxygen by the body; often refers to a measurement of the oxygen requirements.

pectoralis major—Muscle at the upper front chest that extends from the breastbone to the upper arm; it is responsible for pulling the arm across the body.

physiological—Relating to the normal underlying physical and chemical processes within an organism, in this case, humans.

proprioception—The ability to perceive a joint position internally, using sensors within the joints, muscles, and ligaments that surround joints. This information is relayed to the brain, which then modifies muscle activity to accommodate to the joint input.

proprioceptive neuromuscular facilitation (PNF)—Activities that utilize normal reflexes and neural pathways to stimulate additional muscular responses.

quadriceps—Group of four muscles on the front of the thigh. These muscles straighten the knee and also help to flex the hip.

range of motion—The movement available at a joint; often described as active or passive. Full range of motion is the total possible motion in any one plane of movement.

rating of perceived exertion (RPE)—A method of rating the difficulty of an activity, using the individual's perception of the difficulty of the exercise.

rehabilitation—Treatment to restore to normal activities an individual who has been injured or ill.

repetition maximum (RM)—The heaviest weight that can be lifted in a trial. The most common are 1-, 6-, and 10-repetition trials.

rhomboids—These muscles extend from the shoulder blade to the spine and help to pull the shoulder blades toward the center of the body.

splints—Also known as orthotics, these devices help to stabilize or control motion at a joint.

stabilization exercises—Exercises that emphasize isometric-type contractions of the muscles that support the spine.

stiffness—Resistance to fluid motion of a muscle, usually uncomfortable.

synovial fluid—A special fluid that is secreted within most joints. It acts like oil, decreasing friction within the joint during movement.

target heart rate (THR)—Desired exercise heart rate that induces a training response throughout the body.

trapezius—This muscle at the top and back of the shoulder and neck has three parts that help to raise and lower the shoulder blade, as well as pull it toward the spine.

triceps—Muscle on the back of the upper arm; it straightens the elbow and helps extend the shoulder.

Valsalva maneuver—Exhalation against a closed glottis; in other words, holding the breath when the natural instinct would be to let the breath out.

REFERENCES

American College of Sports Medicine. 1995. *ACSM's guidelines for exercise testing and prescription.* 5th ed. Baltimore: Lippincott Williams & Wilkins.

American College of Sports Medicine. 1998. Position stand on: Exercise and physical activity for older adults. *Medicine and Science in Sports and Exercise* 30:992-1008.

American College of Sports Medicine. 1998. Position stand on: Heat and cold illnesses during distance running. *Medicine and Science in Sports and Exercise* 28:i-x.

American College of Sports Medicine. 2000. *ACSM's guidelines for exercise testing and prescription.* 6th ed. Baltimore: Lippincott Williams & Wilkins.

American College of Sports Medicine. 2002. Position stand on: Progression models in resistance training for healthy adults. *Medicine and Science in Sports and Exercise* 34:364-80.

Åstrand, P.O. 1960. Aerobic work capacity in men and women with special reference to age. *Acta Physiologica Scandinavia* 49 (Suppl. 169):1-92.

Åstrand, P.O., and I. Rhyming. 1954. A nomogram for calculation of aerobic capacity (physical fitness) from pulse rate during submaximal work. *Journal of Applied Physiology* 7:218-21.

Austin, S., and S. Laeng. 2003. Yoga. In *Complementary therapies and wellness: Practice essentials for holistic health care.* Edited by Jodi Carlson. Upper Saddle River, NJ: Prentice Hall.

Baker, K.R., M.E. Nelson, D.T. Felson, J.E. Layne, R. Sarno, and R. Roubenoff. 2001. The efficacy of home based progressive strength training in older adults with knee osteoarthritis: A randomized controlled trial. *The Journal of Rheumatology* 28:1655-65.

Bandy, W.D., J.M. Irion, and M. Briggler. 1997. The effect of time and frequency of static stretching on flexibility of the hamstring muscles. *Physical Therapy* 77:1090-96.

Bandy, W.D., J.M. Irion, and M.Briggler. 1998. The effect of static stretch and dynamic range of motion training on the flexibility of the hamstring muscles. *Journal of Orthopaedic and Sports Physical Therapy* 27:295-300.

Beals, C.A., R.M. Lampman, B.F. Banwell, E.M. Braunstein, J.W. Albers, and C.W. Castor. 1985. Measurement of exercise tolerance in patients with rheumatoid arthritis and osteoarthritis. *Journal of Rheumatology* 12:8458-61.

Buckwalter, J.A., and H.J. Mankin. 1997. Articular cartilage. II. Degeneration and osteoarthrosis, repair, regeneration and transplantation. *Journal of Bone and Joint Surgery* 79:612-32.

Byers, P.H. 1985. Effect of exercise on morning stiffness and mobility in patients with rheumatoid arthritis. *Research in Nursing and Health* 8:275-81.

Calder, P.C. 2002. Dietary modification of inflammation with lipids. *Proceedings of the Nutrition Society* 61:345-58.

Chapman, E., H. DeVries, and R. Swezey. 1972. Joint stiffness: Effects of exercise on young and old men. *Journal of Gerontology* 27:218-21.

Clark, H.H. 1973. Adaptations in strength and muscular endurance resulting from exercise. In *Exercise and Sport Sciences Reviews* edited by J. Wilmore 1:73-98.

Cooper, K.H. 1982. *The aerobics program for total well-being.* New York: Bantam Books.

Curtis, C.L., S.G. Rees, J. Cramp, C.R. Flannery, C.E. Hughes, C.B. Little, et al. 2002. Effects of n-3 fatty acids on cartilage metabolism. *Proceedings of the Nutrition Society* 61: 381-89.

Dolgener, F.A., L.D. Hensley, J.J. Marsh, and J.K. Fjelstul. 1994. Validation of the Rockport fitness walking test in college males and females. *Research Quarterly for Exercise and Sport* 65:152-158.

Ekblom, B., O. Lovgren, M. Alderin, M. Fridström, and G. Sätterström. 1974. Physical performance in patients with rheumatoid arthritis. *Scandinavian Journal of Rheumatology* 3:121-25.

Falconer, J.A. 2001. Deconditioning. In *Clinical care in the rheumatic diseases.* 2nd ed. Atlanta: American College of Rheumatology.

Felson, D.T., and Y. Zhang. 1998. An update on the epidemiology of knee and hip osteoarthritis with a view to prevention. *Arthritis and Rheumatism* 41:1342-55.

Felson, D.T., Y. Zhang, J.M. Anthony, A. Niamark, and J.J. Anderson. 1992. Weight loss reduces the risk for symptomatic knee osteoarthritis in women. The Framingham Study. *Annals of Internal Medicine* 116:535-39.

Fries, J.F., G. Singh, D. Morfield, H.B. Hubert, N.E. Lane, and B.W. Brown Jr. 1994. Running and the development of disability with age. *Annals of Internal Medicine* 121:502-9.

Garfinkel, M.S., H.R. Schumacher, A. Hussain, M. Levy, and R.A. Reshetar. 1994. Evaluation of a yoga-based regimen for treatment of osteoarthritis of the hands. *Journal of Rheumatology* 21:2341-43.

Goodman, C.C., and W.G. Boissonnault. 2003. Bone, joint, and soft tissue disorders. In *Pathology: Implications for the physical therapist.* 5th ed. Edited by C.C. Goodman, W.G. Boissonnault, and K.S. Fuller. Philadelphia: Saunders.

Hanes, B. 1996. Orthotics, splinting, and lifestyle factors. In *Physical therapy in arthritis.* Edited by J.M. Walker and A. Helewa. Philadelphia: W.B. Saunders Co.

Hardy, M.A. 1989. The biology of scar formation. *Physical Therapy* 69:1015-24.

Harlowe, D., and P. Yu. 1997. *The ROM DANCE: A range of motion exercise and relaxation program.* Madison, WI: Uncharted Country Publishing.

Hertling, D., and R.M. Kessler. 1996. *Management of common musculoskeletal disorders: Physical therapy principles and methods.* 5th ed. Philadelphia: Lippincott.

Hillstrom, H.J., K. Whitney, J. McGuire, D.J. Brower, C. Riegger-Krugh, and H.R. Schumacher. 2001. Lower extremity conservative realignment therapies and ambulatory aids. In *Clinical care in the rheumatic diseases.* 2nd ed. Atlanta: American College of Rheumatology.

Hillstrom, H.J., K. Whitney, J. McGuire, R.T. Mahan, and H. Lemont. 2001. Evaluation and management of the foot and ankle. In *Clinical care in the rheumatic diseases.* 2nd ed. Atlanta: American College of Rheumatology.

Hoeger, W.W., and S.A. Hoeger. 2002. *Principles and labs for fitness and wellness.* 6th ed. Belmont, CA: Wadsworth/Thomson Learning.

Holten, O. 1993. *Medisinsk treningsterapi.* Oslo: Universitetsforlaget.

Hootman, J. 2002. The burden of arthritis PA and the development of arthritis. Paper presented at the Annual Conference of the American College of Sports Medicine, St. Louis, MO.

Hoppenfeld, S. 1976. *Physical examination of the spine and extremities.* East Norwalk, CT: Appleton-Century-Crofts.

Hurley, B.F., and J.M. Hagberg. 1998. Optimizing health in older persons: Aerobic or strength training? *Exercise and Sport Sciences Reviews* 26:61-89.

Hurley, M.V., D.L. Scott, J. Rees, and D.J. Newham. 1997. Sensorimotor changes and functional performance in patients with knee osteoarthritis. *Annals of Rheumatic Disease* 56:641-48.

Jadelis, K., M.E. Miller, W.H. Ettinger Jr., and S.P. Messier. 2001. Strength, balance, and the modifying effects of obesity and knee pain: Results from the Observational Arthritis Study in Seniors (OASIS). *Journal of the American Geriatrics Society* 49:884-91.

Janis, L.R. 1990. Aerobic dance survey: A study of high-impact versus low-impact injuries. *Journal of the American Podiatry Medical Association* 80:419-23.

Kendall, F.P., E.K. McCreary, and P.G. Provance. 1993. *Muscles testing and function.* 4th ed. Baltimore: Williams & Wilkins.

Kirstein, A., F. Dietz, and S.M. Hwang. 1991. Evaluating the safety and potential use of a weight-bearing exercise, T'ai Chi Chuan, for rheumatoid arthritis patients. *American Journal of Physical Medicine and Rehabilitation.* 70:136-41.

Kisner, C., and L.A. Colby. 2002. *Therapeutic exercise.* 4th ed. Philadelphia: F.A. Davis Company.

Kline, G.M., J.P. Porcari, R. Hintermeister, P.S. Freedson, A.Ward, R.F. McCarron, J. Ross, and J.M. Rippe. 1987. Estimation of $\dot{V}O_2$max from a one-mile track walk, gender, age, and body weight. *Medicine and Science in Sports and Exercise* 19:253-59.

Knight, K.L. 1979. Knee rehabilitation by the daily adjustable progressive resistance exercise program. *American Journal of Sports Medicine* 7:336-1979.

Lan, C., J. Lai, S. Chen, and M. Wong. 1998. Twelve-month t'ai chi training in the elderly: Its effect on health fitness. *Medicine and Science in Sports and Exercise* 30:345-51.

Lane, N.E., D.A. Bloch, P.D. Wood, and J.F. Fries. 1987. Aging, long-distance running, and the development of musculoskeletal disability: A controlled study. *American Journal of Medicine* 82:772-80.

Lieberson, W.T. 1984. Brief isometric exercise. In *Therapeutic exercise.* 4th ed. Edited by J. Basmajian. Baltimore: Williams & Wilkins.

Liu, S.H., and R. Mirzayan. 1995. Current review: Functional knee bracing. *Clinical Orthopaedics* 317:273-81.

Lozada, C.J., and R.R. Altman. 2001. Osteoarthritis. In *Clinical care in the rheumatic diseases.* 2nd ed. Atlanta: American College of Rheumatology.

Lumsden, D.B., A. Baccala, and J. Martire. 1998. T'ai chi for osteoarthritis: An introduction for primary care physicians. *Geriatrics* 53:84, 87-88.

Matsuda, S. 2003. T'ai chi. In *Complementary therapies and wellness: Practice essentials for holistic health care.* Edited by Jodi Carlson. Upper Saddle River, NJ: Prentice Hall.

McArdle, W.D., F.I. Katch, and V.L. Katch. 2000. *Essentials of exercise physiology.* 2nd ed. Baltimore: Lippincott Williams & Wilkins.

McGill, S.M. 2001. Low back stability: From formal description to issues for performance and rehabilitation. *Exercise and Sport Sciences Reviews* 29:26-31.

Minor, M.A. 1991. Physical activity and management of arthritis. *Annals of Behavioral Medicine* 13:117-24.

Minor, M.A. 1996. Cardiovascular health and physical fitness for the client with multiple joint involvement. In *Physical therapy in arthritis.* Edited by J. Walker and A. Helewa. Philadelphia: W.B. Saunders.

Minor, M.A., J.E. Hewett, R.R. Webel, S.K. Anderson, and D.R. Kay. 1989. Efficacy of physical conditioning exercise in patients with rheumatoid arthritis and osteoarthritis. *Arthritis and Rheumatology* 32:1396-1405.

Minor, M.A., and M.D.Westby. 2001. Rest and exercise. In *Clinical care in the rheumatic diseases.* 2nded. Atlanta: American College of Rheumatology.

Morrow, J.R., S.J. FitzGerald, A.W. Jackson, H.R. Bowles, and S.N. Blair. 2002. Relation between 10-year history of physical activity and injury and incidence of osteoarthritis. *Medicine and Science in Sports and Exercise* 34:S156 (abstract).

Müller-Faßbender, H., G.L. Bach, W. Haase, L.C. Rovati, and I. Setnikar. 1994. Glucosamine sulfate compared to ibuprofen in osteoarthritis of the knee. *Osteoarthritis and Cartilage* 2:61-69.

National Academy of Sciences. 2001. *Recommended dietary allowances.* 10th ed. Washington, DC: National Academy Press.

Nichols, L.A. 2001. History and physical assessment. In *Clinical care in the rheumatic diseases.* 2nd ed. Atlanta: American College of Rheumatology,

Noack, W., M. Fischer, K.K. Förster, L.C. Rovati, and I. Setnikar. 1994. Glucosamine sulfate in osteoarthritis. *Osteoarthritis and Cartilage* 2:51-59.

Noreau, L., H. Martineau, L. Roy, and M. Belzile. 1995. Effects of a modified dance-based exercise on cardiorespiratory fitness, psychological state, and health status of persons with rheumatoid arthritis. *American Journal of Physical Rehabilitation* 74:19-27.

Noreau, L., H. Moffet, M. Drolet, and E. Parent. 1997. Dance-based exercise program in rheumatoid arthritis: Feasibility in individuals with American College of Rheumatology functional class III disease. *American Journal of Physical Rehabilitation* 76:109-13.

Panush, R.S., and D.G. Brown. 1987. Exercise in arthritis. *Sports Medicine* 4:54-64.

Pate, R.R., M.M. Pratt, S.N. Blair, W.L. Haskell, C.A. Macera, C. Bouchard, et al. 1995. Physical activity and public health: A recommendation from the Centers for Disease Control and Prevention and the American College of Sports Medicine. *Journal of the American Medical Association* 273:402-7.

Perlman, S.G., K.J. Connell, A. Clark, M.S. Robinson, P. Conlon, M. Gecht, P. Caldron, and J.M. Sinacore. 1990. Dance-based aerobic exercise for rheumatoid arthritis. *Arthritis Care* 3:29-35.

Pollock, M.L., G.A. Gaesser, J.D. Butcher, J.P. Despres, R.K. Dishman, B.A. Franklin, and C. Ewing-Garber. 1998. American College of Sports Medicine: The recommended quantity and quality of exercise for developing and maintaining cardiorespiratory and muscular fitness, and flexibility in healthy adults. *Medicine and Science in Sports and Exercise* 30:975-91.

Prochaska, J.O., and C.C. DiClemente. 1982. Transtheoretical therapy: Toward a more integrative model of change. *Psychotherapy: Theory, Research, and Practice* 19:276-288.

Qui, X.G., S.N. Gao, G. Giacovelli, L. Rovati, and I. Setnikar. 1998. Efficacy and safety of glucosamine sulfate versus ibuprofen in patients with knee osteoarthritis. *Arzneimittel-Forschung Drug Research* 48:469-74.

Reginster, J.Y., R. Deroisy, L.C. Rovati, R.L. Lee, E. Lejeune, O. Bruyere, et al. 2001. Long-term effects of glucosamine sulphate on osteoarthritis progression: A randomized, placebo-controlled clinical trial. *Lancet* 357:251-56.

Robertson, R.J., and B.J. Noble. 1997. Perception of physical exertion: Methods, mediators, and applications. *Exercise and Sport Sciences Reviews,* edited by J. Holloszy 25:407-52.

Rogers, M.A., and W.J. Evans. 1993. Changes in skeletal muscle with aging: Effects of exercise training. *Exercise and Sport Sciences Reviews* 21:65-102.

Rothenberger, L.A., J.I. Chang, and T.A. Cable. 1988. Prevalence and types of injuries in aerobic dancers. *American Journal of Sports Medicine* 16:403-7.

Sady, S.P., M. Wortman, and D. Blanke. 1982. Flexibility training: Ballistic, static or proprioceptive neuromuscular facilitation? *Archives of Physical Medicine and Rehabilitation* 63:261-63.

Sale, D.G. 1988. Neural adaptation to resistance training. *Medicine and Science in Sports and Exercise* 20 (Suppl.):135-45.

Sanford-Smith, S., M. MacKay-Lyons, and S. Nunes-Clement. 1998. Therapeutic benefit of aquaerobics for individuals with rheumatoid arthritis. *Physiotherapy Canada* 50: 40-46.

Sapega, A.A., T.C. Quendenfeld, R.A. Moyer, and R.A. Butler. 1981. Biophysical factors in range of motion exercise. *Physician and Sportsmedicine* 9:57-65.

Sharma, L., J. Song, D.T. Felson, S. Cahae, E. Shamiyeh, and D.D. Dunlop. 2001. The role of knee alignment in disease progression and functional decline in knee osteoarthritis. *Journal of the American Medical Association* 286:188-95.

Stamford, B.A. 1988. Exercise and the elderly. *Exercise and Sports Sciences Reviews* 16: 341-79.

Suomi, R., and S. Lindauer. 1997. Effectiveness of Arthritis Foundation Aquatic Program on strength and range of motion in women with arthritis. *Journal of Aging and Physical Activity* 5:341-52.

Suter, E., and W. Herzog. 2000. Does muscle inhibition after knee injury increase the risk of osteoarthritis? *Exercise and Sport Sciences Reviews* 28:15-23.

Tidow-Kebritchi, S., and S. Mobarhan. 2001. Effects of diets containing fish oil and vitamin E on rheumatoid arthritis. *Nutrition Reviews* 59:335-38.

U.S. Department of Health and Human Services. 1996. *Physical activity and health: A report of the Surgeon General.* Atlanta: Centers for Disease Control and Prevention, National Center for Chronic Disease Prevention and Health Promotion.

U.S. Department of Health and Human Services, Department of Agriculture. 2000. Nutrition and your health: Dietary guidelines for Americans. *Home and Garden Bulletin* No. 232. Washington DC: Department of Health and Human Services.

Westby, M.D. 2001. A health professional's guide to exercise prescription for people with arthritis: A review of aerobic fitness activities. *Arthritis Care Research* 45:501-11.

Whaley, M.H., and L.A. Kaminisky. 2001. Epidemiology of physical activity, physical fitness, and selected chronic diseases. In *ACSM's resource manual for guidelines for exercise testing and prescription.* 4th ed. Baltimore: Lippincott Williams & Wilkins.

Wharton, J., and P. Wharton. 1996. *The Whartons' stretch book.* New York: Times Book/ Random House.

Wrightson, J.D., and G.A. Malanga. 2001. Strengthening and other therapeutic exercise in the treatment of osteoarthritis. *Physical Medicine and Rehabilitation: State of the Art Reviews* 15:43-56.

Young, D.R., J. Appel, J. SunHa, and E.R. Miller. 1999. The effects of aerobic exercise and T'ai Chi on blood pressure in older people: Results of a randomized trial. *Journal of the American Geriatric Society* 47:277-84.

INDEX

Note: The italicized *f* and *t* following page numbers refer to figures and tables, respectively.

ABOUT THE AUTHOR

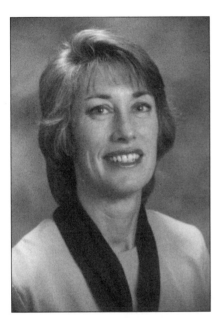

A. Lynn Millar, PT, PhD, FACSM, is professor of physical therapy and assistant program chair in the department of physical therapy at Andrews University. She received her PhD in exercise physiology at Arizona State University. She specializes in therapeutic exercise for several conditions including arthritis. Her areas of research include work with track athletes, injury prevention and treatment, and other therapy-related topics.

Millar first joined the American College of Sports Medicine (ACSM) in 1978 and has been a fellow of the ACSM since 1992. She has been involved extensively in the Midwest Regional Chapter of the ACSM, having served as the president as well as serving on the Communications and Public Information and Membership committees. She is also a member of the American Physical Therapy Association. Millar has served as a manuscript reviewer for the *Journal of Orthopaedic and Sports Physical Therapy* (JOSPT) and ACSM's flagship journal, *Medicine & Science in Sport & Exercise* (MSSE).

Millar lives in Granger, Indiana, and enjoys playing golf, running, and reading.

ABOUT THE ACSM

The **American College of Sports Medicine** (ACSM) is dedicated to promoting healthier lifestyles for people around the globe through scientific research, education, and the practical application of knowledge in sports medicine and exercise science. The ACSM has more than 20,000 international, national, and regional members in 80 countries who work in a range of medical specialties, allied health professions, and scientific disciplines. This diversity and expertise make the ACSM the largest, most-respected sports medicine and exercise science organization in the world.